Mimea Press, 3323 NE 33rd Ave, Portland, Oregon 97212

Getting to Know Clinic HQ
Clemmer, Gina N.

ISBN-13: 978-0615820712 (Mimea Publishing)

The information in this document is subject to change without notice. Errata for this document can be located at www.clinichq.org.

Getting to know CLINICHQ

A Message from the Executive Director

Operating a spay/neuter clinic is a labor of love. It's so wonderful to help animals every day. It's an honor to work with dedicated and smart people, who also believe as I do, that spay/neuter can change the world.

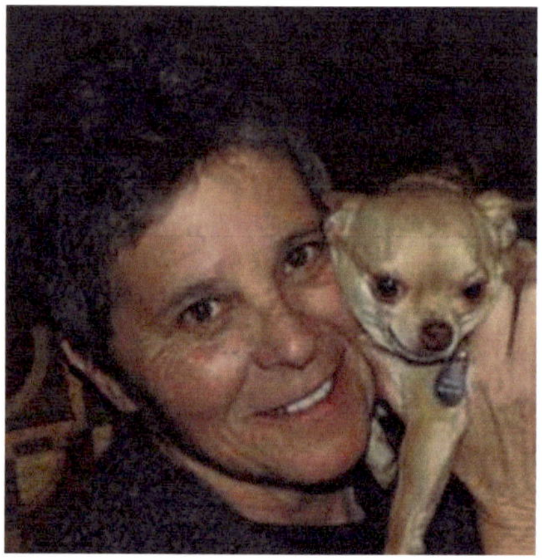

Then there is the data, entering it, managing it, using it. When Humane Alliance first opened, we made appointments with a pen and paper in a big book at the front desk. We've learned a lot in nineteen years. Also in that time, the world has changed.

Numeric data is expected from funders to get and keep funding. We can analyze our population in a more sophisticated and detailed way. We can now even pull up a real time map of all the animals we've sterilized within seconds. We use data every single day at Humane Alliance. It has been a challenge in our journey to manage that data, which is why we created Clinic HQ.

We've spent the past year analyzing workflows and counting mouse clicks to create a simple but sophisticated software, tailored to the particular needs of high volume, spay/neuter clinics. Although there is more work to do, I believe we've created a clinic management software that meets the needs of today, and provides a strong foundation for whatever we meet on the horizon.

Sincerely,

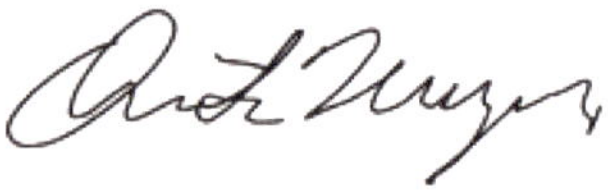

Quita Mazzina

Thank you for choosing Clinic HQ as your clinic management solution. We hope you are ready to save time and accurately record data, so you can better serve your clients and community.

In this comprehensive manual we will give you step by step instructions for each and every function in Clinic HQ. Our goal is to make this already extremely user friendly program even easier to navigate. This manual will walk you through each process in the same order as your work flow, so you won't have to guess what's next. Plus, we will give you extra tips and shortcuts, so you can maximize your productivity.

Each chapter is a direct reflection of its matching colorful icon at the top of your Clinic HQ home page. Think of each icon as a door to a room where you will be able to perform different functions. For example: you will be able to apply payments, bill clients, and print invoices under the green accounting icon. We will use these colorful icons throughout the manual as visual cues, so what you see in the manual will match where you are in the program.

Technical Specifications

Clinic HQ is web-based, so you don't need any fancy equipment to run it. It is mobile ready and optimized for tablets, so you can even run Clinic HQ in your mobile van! Google Chrome is the preferred browser. You can download Google Chrome for free on any computer with an internet connection.

Log in to Clinic HQ and Get Started Now!

1. Enter clinichq.org into your web browser (it does not matter if you type in www. or not)
2. Enter your username and password into the open fields and click <Log In>
   Note: Your user name will be your clinic e-mail address, and you will receive an e-mail with instructions on how to set up your password

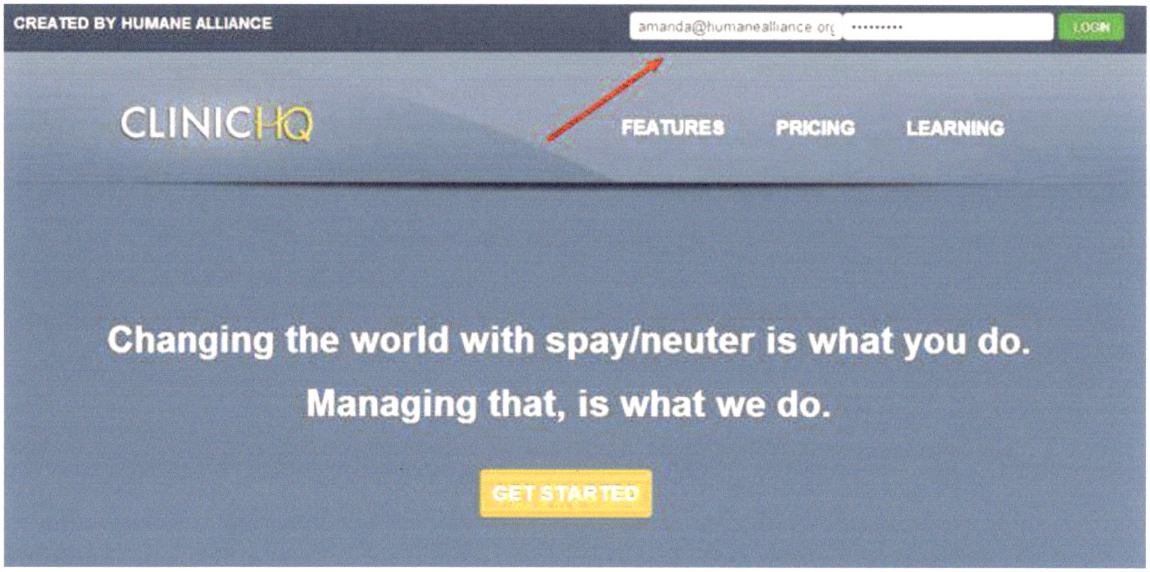

Chapter

1

Dashboard

The Clinic HQ Dashboard will give you a daily snapshot of today's appointments broken into three status bars; appointments pending, in progress, and daily count (number checked out). Color coding allows you to view current status with a single glance, so you know what the day holds in store for your clinic. Dashboard is also equipped with a centrally located search field, for your convenience. Plus, enjoy a nifty IM function so that you and your co-workers stay connected! So what's on your Dashboard? Let's dig a little deeper.

- Daily Snapshot
- Search Feature
- IM Function

Daily Snapshot

Pending: The yellow bar reflects the number of appointments that are scheduled for today. It will decline throughout the day as animals are checked in.

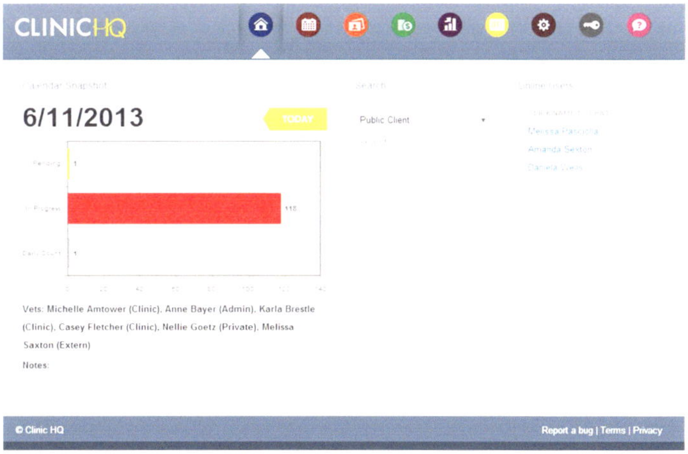

In Progress: The red bar shows the number of animals in clinic. This bar will appear after animals begin to check in and the first round of paperwork is entered.

Daily Count: The grey bar represents the number of animals that have been checked out for the day. It will not appear until animals have been completely processed and checked out.

Vets: Vets on staff for that day will display below your daily snapshot. For clinics with multiple vets performing different functions, this is particularly helpful.

Notes: Clinic wide notes will be displayed on your Dashboard as well. This feature can be used for important announcements that all users will need to know for that day. For example, if a specific voucher has expired and is no longer valid at your clinic, you can enter that information here. The user must have permission to add these notes in their Clinic HQ user profile, so that not just anyone can add an important note. We will show you where to enter these notes in Chapter 2.

Search Feature

This quick search feature is conveniently located to the right of your daily snapshot. You can search by the following categories with the drop down menu on your Dashboard.

- Public Client Name
- Volume Client Name
- Volume Client Owner Name
- Animal #
- Animal Name
- Microchip
- Rabies tag

After selecting from the drop down menu, simply enter the first three letters or numbers of your search into the field below it and hit enter. A list of names will generate below it. Select from the list and your search is complete!

IM Function

To the far right of your Dashboard screen, you will see a box for instant messaging with co-workers. When someone's name appears in that box, it means they are online and available to receive IMs from you. Click on the person's name you wish to chat with. This will open a small message box. Type your message and hit enter to send. When someone sends you a message, the top of your text box will blink orange. Click on the person's name you are messaging with to minimize the chat box. This will allow you to chat with multiple users at the same time. Use these fun, colorful emoticons in your messages as an added bonus!

IM Function is for interoffice use only.
IM messages are confidential and cannot be viewed by other co-workers.

Report a Bug

If you encounter a system issue while using Clinic HQ, you can report a bug from any page of the software. In the bottom right hand corner of every screen, there is a <Report a Bug> link. When you select this link, it will capture your current screen, and give you a pop up box so you can describe the error in the description field. Select <Send Report> button to automatically send an e-mail with this information to our technical support team, so that it can be repaired as quickly as possible.

Chapter 2

Calendar

The Calendar section of Clinic HQ is your one stop shop for making all public, volume, and recheck appointments. You are also able to view and adjust capacity by the day, week, and month in this section! Below is a brief overview of what we will cover in this Chapter.

- Calendar at a glance – Features & Functions
- Calendar Anatomy
- Making Appointments
    - Public
    - Volume
    - Recheck

Calendar at a Glance – Features & Functions

The Calendar has many helpful features & functions that will allow you to organize your clinic's appointments quickly and easily, but there are few things you need to know first.

Color Coded Capacity: This feature makes it easy to see which days are busier than others, thus providing a quick reference when making new appointments. Capacity management variables can be adjusted by the day here as well. We will go into more detail in ***Chapter 7*** on how to set your clinic's daily capacity.

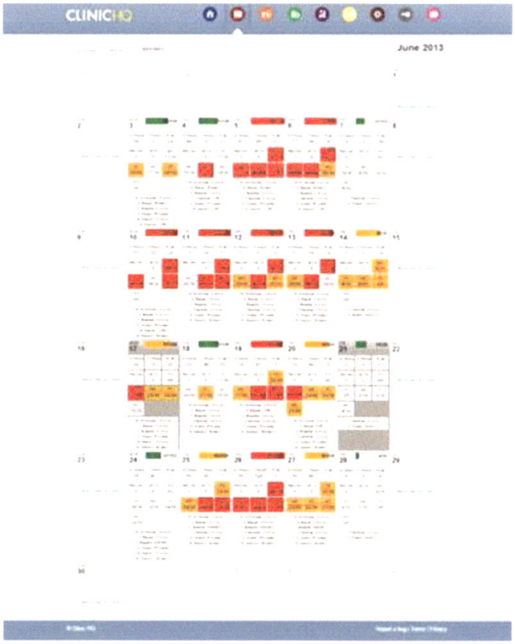

Color Coded Capacity: GREEN – Clinic is below 70% capacity (plenty of appointments available); Orange – Clinic is at 70% capacity; RED – clinic is at 90% capacity or higher.

Detailed Monthly Appointment View: The color coded tiles on the monthly calendar also show how many patients and what type of patients are scheduled for each day of the month. For a more detailed view of each day's appointments, click on the day you want to view.

Calendar Drop Down Menu: This feature, located to the right of the default month tab in Calendar, gives you the option of clicking on what you would like to see displayed on your monthly view. For example: If you only wanted to view appointments for female cats coming in on self transport, you could deselect the rest of the boxes in the drop down menu and be left with only this information.

This preference is specific to each user. So if it benefits your position at the clinic to only view certain tiles, you only have to set them once!

Quickly Reopen a Closed Day: Click on the blue <mark day as open> link on any day marked closed on the monthly view. Select YES when the window opens and asks if you would like to re-open the day.

Weekly View: The <This Week> tab to the left of the default monthly view gives you an even better breakdown of your daily events for the week. This tab allows you to enter notes for each day that will display on your Dashboard beneath the Daily Snapshot. It also provides you with a tool for adjusting capacity, vet type, and for marking a clinic day closed.

***To Enter Notes*:** Type note in the text box for the selected day. Then click the green check box to the right of the note to save it. (This will now show up on all users Dashboards on that day!) Note: Since notes are clinic wide, you must have permission to do this in your user profile.

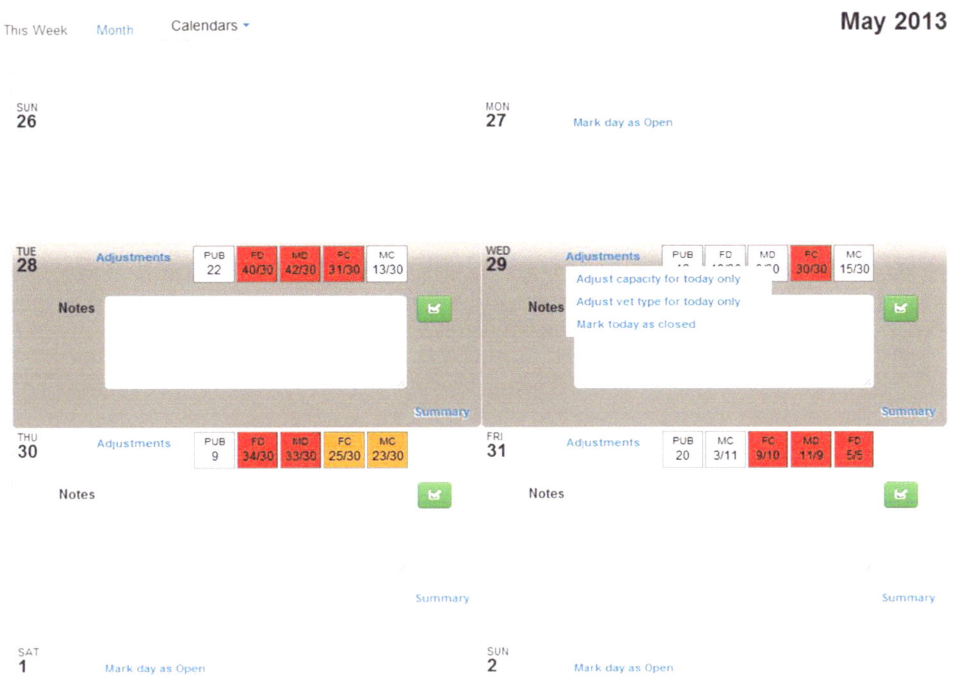

Adjustments: Hover over the blue "adjustments" link that is located on each day of your weekly view. This will give you three options: Adjust Capacity for Today Only, Adjust Vet Type for Today Only, and Mark Today as Closed.

To Adjust Capacity: Click on blue link titled <Adjust Capacity for Today Only> in the list under <Adjustments>. This will bring up another window. You will notice that if you hover over the page, the only places where you can enter information will be under the heading Daily Max. From here you can adjust these numbers based on your clinic's ability to perform these types of surgeries for that particular day.

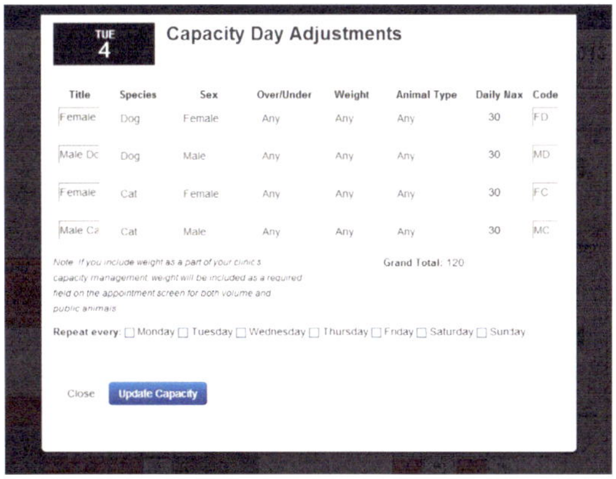

Have 1 vet most days of the week, but 2 vets on Thursdays and Fridays? Check the boxes at the bottom of your Capacity Adjustment screen, so that your adjusted capacity repeats for those days of the week, every week!

To Adjust Vet Type: For clinics with multiple vets performing different duties, this function is particularly helpful. Click on the blue link titled <Adjust Vet Type for Today Only>.

Another window will pop up with all of the vets and their function for the day listed. From here you can enter the new vet type to the right of their name and save.

To Mark Today as Closed: Click on the blue link titled <Mark Today as Closed> and another window will pop up. From here you will be able to enter a description of the closing. You will not be able to adjust the date, because the function is to close the clinic for today. Click <Closed Appointment> to save your change.

*__Move on to Next Week or Month__: To move your calendar on to the next month or week, simply click on the last day on the displayed calendar showing no activity. This will automatically take you to next month or week. To go back, click on the first day of the calendar showing no activity and the previous month or week will be displayed.

Calendar Anatomy

The Calendar might look strange to you when you first begin using Clinic HQ. Learn how to read the Clinic HQ calendar in this section, so you get the most out of this function.

What does each tile stand for on the Calendar?

Each tile on the calendar stands for a specific type of appointment.

Humane Alliance breaks their calendar down into the four main types of surgeries, transport types, and recheck appointments for example. You can set your user profile to see only what you want to see, and can change it at any time with the Calendar drop down menu.

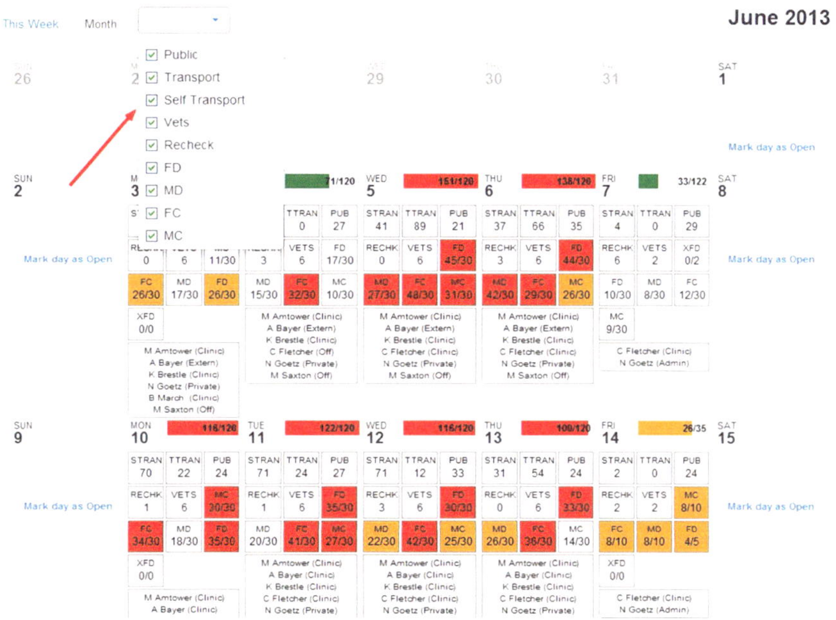

The codes on each tile are created in Settings > Capacity Management. Example codes may include FD for Female Dog, or MC for Male Cat.

Each tile is color coded so it is easy for volunteers and staff to see when one type of surgery has met its capacity for the day, and that they should look for another day to book

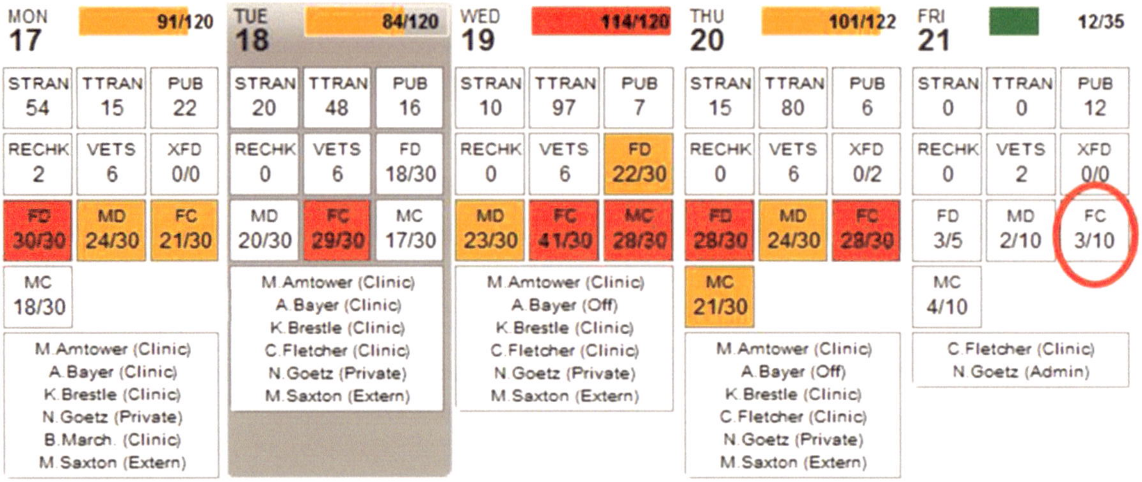

You see how on the rest of the days of the week, the FC tiles are in red, and at or over capacity? Friday would be the best day to book a female cat surgery.

What do the numbers mean on the Calendar?

The numbers at the top of each Calendar day, in the status bar, stand for the total number appointments as compared to the set total capacity for that day. The status bar is color coded as well, so you can see when your clinic has reached its total capacity for that day.

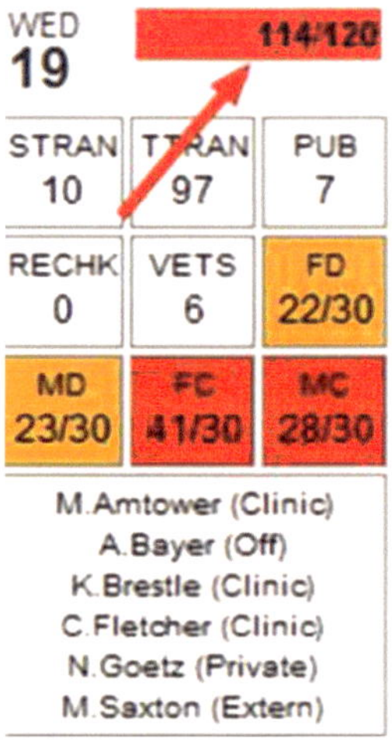

Total Appointments/Total Capacity

The numbers on each tile are similar in that they are the total numbers of each individual category. For categories with set capacity, the second number will be the set capacity for that category on that day.

Ex: Number of Female Cat Appointments/Set Capacity for Female Cat Surgeries

You will notice that Clinic HQ will not prevent you from overbooking appointments, even if you have met your capacity. We have left this option available to provide more flexibility in the event of no shows.

***Bonus Recheck Appointment Calendar Feature**

When you hover over the Recheck tile on your calendar, a small list of all of your rechecks and their appointment times will appear! Need a quick glance? Hover and done!

Making Appointments

Clinic HQ's Calendar is your appointment making hub! This section will be divided into three specific types of appointment making and we will tell you how to perform each of these functions in detail. Note: Volume clients are the organizations that you have special relationships with like shelters and rescue groups.

- Make Public Appointment
- Make Volume Client Appointment
- Make Recheck Appointment

Make Public Appointment

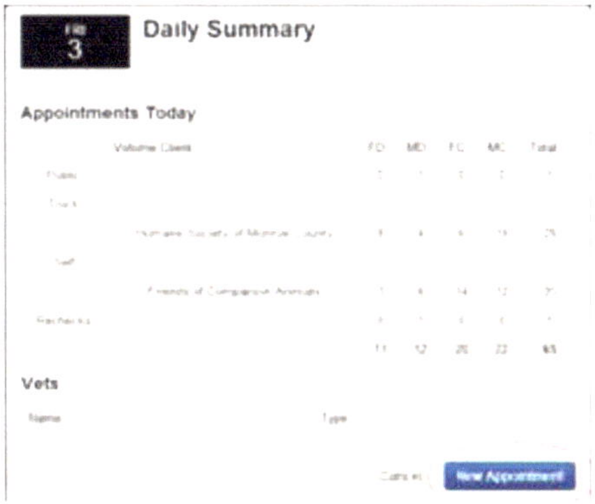

1. Gather client and animal details
2. Click on <Calendar> Icon
3. Identify available date tile from the month view calendar and click on it

4. Daily Summary pop up box will now appear
5. Click on <New Appointment> button at the bottom right of the box
6. Another data box will appear
7. Confirm appointment date, and change on this screen if necessary
8. Select <Spay or Neuter> from drop down menu next to appointment type
9. Select <Public> from client type drop down menu, this will make public fields visible
10. Fill in client details. Anything with an * is a required field.

Tips: *If the client has visited your clinic before, their information will automatically populate after you enter the first three letters of their last name. If the populated name is not correct, click outside of the pop up box and continue to enter manually.*

The address must be correct for the client. *Google Maps is working while you are to pinpoint a location that will be used for geographic data and reports. If you cannot get the address you have received from the client to work, enter the clinic's address to move forward.*

11. Click on Animal button/tab at the bottom or top of the page
12. Enter animal details. Anything with an *is a required field

Tips: *For animal years enter 0 if animal is under 1 year of age. If client does not know the animal's age by the month over 1 year old enter 0 for the month. It is required to enter both animal's year and month of age.*

13. Select animal's primary breed from the drop down menu. *Note: If the species is a mix select the mix box in addition to the primary breed. If you do not know the primary breed select unknown from the drop down menu and then select the mix box.*

14. If client requests additional services or products (ex: a rabies vaccine, nail trim) click on the blue link <Services and Products> in the upper right corner of the animal detail box.
15. Enter the quantity of each additional service or product the client has requested and click the <Save> button.
16. Click <Clone> button on the bottom right of the animal tab screen to enter mul tiple animals for one client!
17. Repeat the above process for each animal
18. Click the summary tab to the right of the animal tab to view appointment details
19. Click <Make Appointment> button at the bottom of the screen to complete
20. Click <Make and Checkout> if the client is a walk in (same day)

Make Volume Client Appointment

1. Click on <Calendar> Icon
2. Identify available date tile from the month view calendar and click
3. Daily Summary pop up box will now appear
4. Click on <New Appointment> button at the bottom right of the box
5. Another data box will appear
6. Confirm appointment date, and change on this screen if necessary

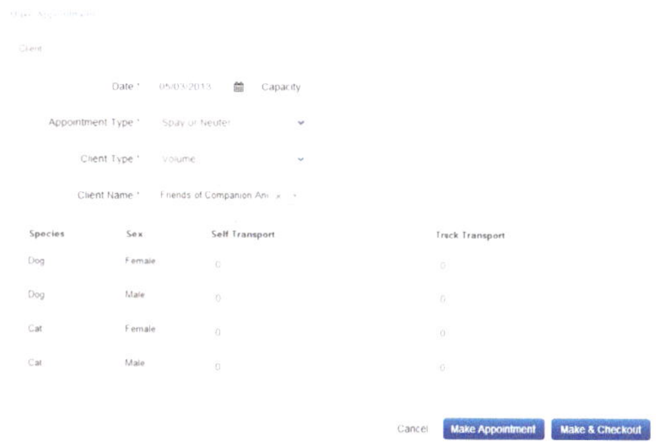

7. Select Spay or Neuter from drop down menu next to appointment type
8. Select Volume from client type drop down menu, this will make volume fields visible

9. Search for Volume client name Note:
   All Volume Clients much be set up in the system prior to making appointments. We will teach you how to Create Volume Clients in **Chapter 3**
10. Enter the numbers of each type of animal in the designated fields. *Note: Some clients may be self transport (the client delivers the animals) and some may be truck transport (your clinic picks up the animals) you can make this distinction*
11. Click <Make Appointment> button at the bottom of the page to save

Make Recheck Appointment

1. Click on <Calendar> Icon
2. Identify available date tile from the month view calendar and click on it
3. Daily Summary pop up box will now appear
4. Click on <New Appointment> button at the bottom right of the box
5. Another data box will appear
6. Confirm appointment date, and change on this screen if necessary
7. Select <Recheck> from drop down menu next to appointment type
8. Select client type from drop down menu (volume or public)

Note: If the animal was originally brought in by a volume client, you must search by that volume client first. Then search for the animal by name.

9. Enter the first three letters of the client's name in the search field
10. Names will begin to populate below the search field
11. Select the correct name from the list
12. Time and Animal fields will now appear
13. Select time for the recheck appointment

14. Select which animal will be receiving the recheck from the drop down menu
15. Click the <Make Appointment> button to complete or <Make and Checkout> if client is a walk in (same day)

We will show you how to delete, mark as no show, and edit appointments in **Chapter 3**

Chapter

3

Clients

The Clients section of Clinic HQ is the next step in our process. So far you have reviewed your day and made upcoming appointments. Clients is where you will check animals into clinic, check them out at the end of the day, create volume clients and quickly adjust their appointments, and print helpful reports for your staff's use. This chapter will be broken down into the following functions:

- Search Client History
- Create Volume Clients
- Adjust Volume Client Appointments
- Delete and Mark as No Show – Public Appointments
- Process Checkout
- Generate and Print Rabies Certificates
- Quick Entry – Complete Checkout
- Alternate Complete Checkout
- Print Transport & Recheck Lists for Staff Use

Search Client History

This function is used to find any client that has ever done business with your clinic. It will contain the client's personal profile, previous appointments by date, animals listed under that client, and any surgery details that you may need to access after the animal has checked out. Here's how to do it and what you will find!

Public Client: Individuals bringing their owned animals in for surgery
Volume Client: Shelters, rescue groups, or other organizations that bring you large numbers of animals
Volume Client Owner: These animals have actual owners, but are brought in by a volume client

1. Click on <Clients> Icon
2. Select <Search Clients> link from the left hand menu under clients
3. Select type of client from the drop down menu: Public, Volume, or Volume Client Owner
4. Enter first 4 letters of your search in the box to the right of the client type
5. You should now see the client you searched for in a generated list
6. Click on the <View> button to the far right of your client's name
7. Four tabs will now appear in a client details box left to right
8. The General tab is the client's personal data. You can edit this info here and save.

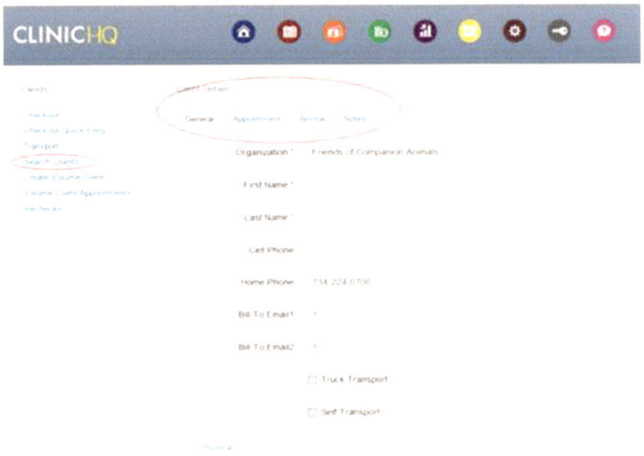

9. The next tab is Appointment. This will show the client's past and present appointments.
10. To reschedule or cancel a current ap pointment, click on the desired button to the right
11. The next tab is <Animal> This will display any animal associated with the client
12. View Summary or Edit Animal details by selecting the desired button to the right
13. Regenerate or Print the animal's rabies certificate by selecting the Rabies button
14. Press print, regenerate, or delete certificate at the bottom of the rabies pop up box
15. The final tab under the client details page is Notes
16. You can enter or review any notes associated with the client under this tab

Create Volume Clients

Before you can even make an appointment for a Volume client, you have to create a profile for them under the Calendar section of Clinic HQ. The ability to have a pre-set profile for this type of client makes appointment making easier, and billing a snap. Let's get started!

1. Click on <Clients> Icon
2. Select <Create Volume Client> link from the left hand main menu
3. Fill in the fields with the primary contact person's information
4. Enter at least one phone number
5. Enter e-mail where invoices can be sent for billing
6. Enter physical, mailing, and billing addresses for client.
7. If all are the same check the <use physical address> box for mailing and billing sections
8. Click <Save Changes> to create volume client

Adjust Volume Client Appointments

After you have made appointments for volume clients in Calendar, you can go to the Client section to quickly adjust these appointments. You can change the patient types, numbers, or how they will be transported right here. This will prevent you from having to delete numerous appointments on the day they are scheduled, or mark them as no shows, which will negatively affect your no show statistics.

1. Click <Clients> Icon
2. Select <Volume Client Appointments> link from the left hand main menu
3. Enter the date of the appointment you would like to adjust
4. A list of the volume clients with appointments for that day will generate

5. To the right of the volume client's appointment you wish to adjust click <edit>
6. Change the numbers in the boxes to reflect the changes you want to make

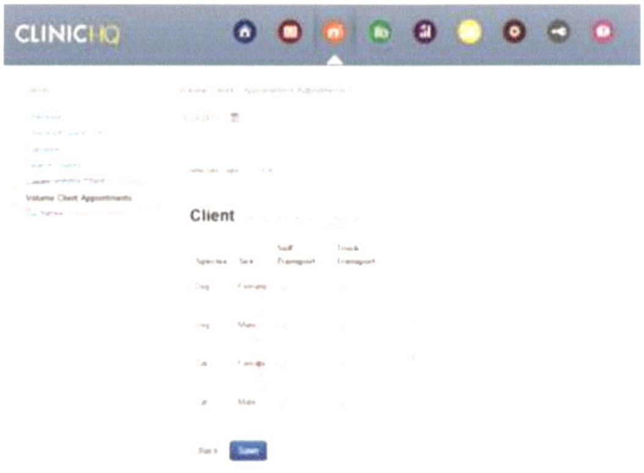

7. Click the <Save> button at the bottom of the box to make the adjustment
8. Click the <Bulk> tab on this page if you need make repeat orders for this client
9. Fill in the boxes with the numbers and types of animals
10. Select the repeating dates that these transports will happen from the calendar under bulk appointments and click the blue <Add> button after selecting each date.
11. The dates will appear bulleted to the right of the animal boxes when they are added
12. Click the green <Bulk Now> button at the bottom of the page to save

Delete Volume Client Appointment

1. Go back to <Volume Client Appointments> link on left hand main menu
2. Enter the date of the appointment you would like to delete
3. A list of volume client appointments for that date will generate
4. Select <Delete All> button to the far right of the volume client's name

Delete and Mark as No Show - Public Appointments

1. Click on <Client> Icon

2. Click on blue <Checkout> link from the left hand main menu
3. A list of all of your appointments for that day will generate.
4. You can change the date at the top of the screen, to delete an upcoming appointment
5. To the right of the name, check the box to delete or mark as no show.
   Note: Use the delete button for duplicate appointments, so you do not affect your record of no shows. Use the delete button as well, if the client called and let you know that they would not be coming in.

Process Checkout

Once animals begin to check in to the clinic for the day, you will begin your checkout process with the first round of paperwork that you receive from the front desk. Any pre-payment will be entered at this time, as well as any client or animal detail corrections. Once you click the start link under checkout, an animal ID will be generated, and the system will know that the animal is now in clinic and being prepped for surgery. You will also generate and print rabies certificates at this time. Let's show you how!

1. Gather your stack of admission forms from the front desk
2. Click on the Client Icon
3. Select <Checkout> link from the left hand main menu
4. All of the appointments for today will be displayed
5. If you need to narrow your search, use the drop down menus at the top of the page

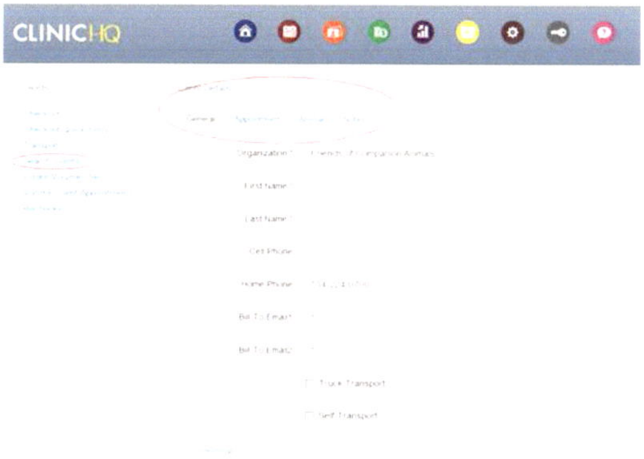

6. Clients with appointments who have not checked in are pending
7. Match the name on the admission form with one on the generated list
8. Click the blue <START> link to the far right of your client's name under status
   Note: This will generate an animal ID and change pending status to in progress.
9. The checkout page with four tabs at the top will now appear
10. The default tab will show the client's details. Check to make sure your paperwork matches what is in the system for the client. Edit if necessary and don't forget to save.
11. Click on the <Animal> tab along the top of the page
12. Enter as much information as you have at this time. Remember any field with an * is required. *Note: For animal years enter 0 if animal is under 1 year of age. If client does not know the animal's age by the month over 1 year old enter 0. Both of these fields are required.*
13. Under animal type use drop down menu to specify whether animal is owned, sheltered, or fostered
14. Click the <Save> button before you move on to the next tab
15. Click on <Services & Products> tab to the right of the animal tab to add addition al services or products (ex: rabies vaccine, nail trim, etc.)
16. Click on the <+> box to the far right of the product or service to add
17. Enter the quantity in the designated box
18. Subsidy (discount) options that may apply for this client will now appear under the subsidy column. We will go over how to set up subsidies in **Chapter 7**.
19. Click on the <+> button under subsidies to view the available discounts for that service
20. Click the blue <+> button in the pop up box to add the subsidy to this client's order
21. Click on the <Financial Tab> to the right of the <Services & Products> tab

22. Enter any cash or check payments on this page
23. For check payments, enter the check number to the right of the payment box
24. Click the blue <Make Payment> button to save
25. Scroll to the bottom of the page to view the updated balance
26. The last step in this process will be to print the rabies certificate

Generate and Print Rabies Certificates

Once all of the information is complete for the first checkout round, a rabies certificate can be generated and printed for the animal. If you are missing any information at this point the system will give you an error message and tell you what is missing, before it will allow you to generate the certificate.

1. Click on the <Rabies Certificate> tab under the Checkout screen
2. This tab only appears if the client requested a rabies vaccine for their animal
3. Click on the <Generate and Print Rabies Certificate> button
4. All details will populate automatically
5. <Print> the certificate to give to the client when they pick up their animal
6. <Regenerate> the certificate if you need an additional copy for your records
7. <Delete> the certificate, if the patient is not given the rabies vaccine and the certificate had already been generated

Print a rabies certificate in 2 seconds or less!
Click Generate and Print Button
Hit enter to print!

*Quick Entry - Complete Checkout

Once your vet has completed surgery on all of the animals in clinic you will receive your final round of paperwork. This is when you complete the checkout process. All of these animals have traveled from a pending status to an in progress status up to this point. Now you will actually check them out. This one page edit screen gets you in and out of your final checkout process!

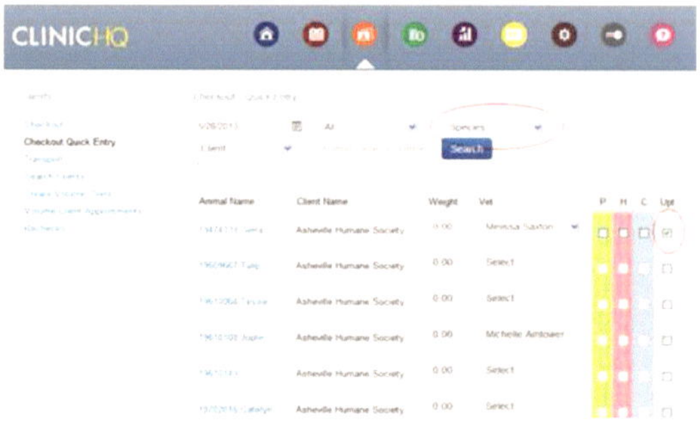

1. Click on the <Client> Icon
2. Click on the blue <Checkout Quick Entry> link on the left hand main menu
3. This will generate a list of all of the animals in clinic
4. You can narrow your list by choosing from the species drop down box
5. Choose the animal you would like to check out from the list
6. Click the check box under the <Upt> (Update) column to activate the row
   Note: Unless you check this Upt box next to the animal you want to edit, you will be unable to make any changes.
7. Input the weight, change the vet, and check any of the three boxes that apply
   Note Color Code: Pregnant is green, In Heat is pink, and Cryptorchid is blue
8. Scroll to the bottom of the page and click the blue <Update> button to check out
   Note: This is very important, because if you navigate away from this page without clicking the update button, your work will not be saved.
9. If the animal requires additional updates to its record, click on the blue link for the animal name and you will be taken back to the original checkout tabs. From there you can enter any additional updates to the animal record.

Alternate Complete Checkout

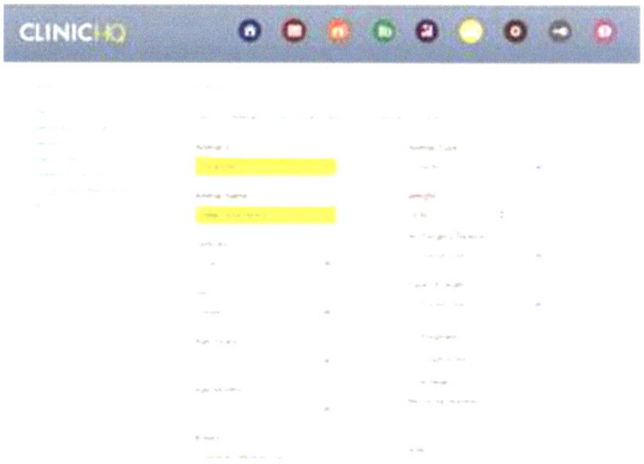

1. Click on the Client Icon
2. Select <Checkout> link from the left hand main menu
3. Change the pending drop down box to <In Progress>
4. You will see a generated list of all animals currently in clinic
5. Click on the blue <In Progress> link to the far right of the chosen animal
6. You will now see all of the tabs you filled in during the first round of checkout
7. Click on the <Animal> tab
8. You will now input the animal's actual weight; the vet who performed the surgery; and whether or not the animal was pregnant, in heat, or cryptorchid
9. Click the <Save> button at the bottom of the page
10. Click on the <Products & Services> tab
11. If any necessary services were added during surgery add these here and review
12. Click the <Financial> tab
13. Review client's balance to see if any additional funds are owed
14. Click the <Details> tab
15. From the drop down menus update the results of any tests or exploratory surgeries performed on the animal (ex: heartworm test, FIV test, etc.)
16. Click the blue <Save> button
17. If all information has been updated, click the green <Checkout> button!

Print Transport and Recheck Lists for Staff Use

Use Clinic HQ's transport list as an end of the day roll call, so your staff knows which animals should go back on which truck. Plus, print a helpful recheck list, so you know how many animals will be revisiting the clinic today. The Client Section of Clinic HQ allows you to print these two convenient reports all in one place.

Print Transport List

1. Click on the Client Icon
2. Click on the blue Transport link from the left hand main menu
3. Today's date will auto fill. You can change it at the top of the page if you wish.
4. A list by volume client with transport will then generate
5. Click on the view button to the far right of the Volume Client
6. Right click with your mouse on the generated report and select <Print>

Print Recheck List

1. Click on the <Client> Icon
2. Click on the blue <Rechecks> link from the left hand main menu
3. Today's scheduled recheck appointments will be displayed
4. Select the <Print PDF List> button to print list

Chapter

4

Accounting

In this section of Clinic HQ you will manage all financial transactions following the checkout process. Apply and adjust payments for both public and volume clients, and view any unpaid balances through the pickup balance list and invoice features. View all item sales for any selected date and balance the day's books with our handy Reconciliation Report! Here is a breakdown of what we will cover in this chapter:

- Public Client Transactions
  - Print Pickup Balance List
  - Apply Payments
- Volume Client Transactions
  - Bill Volume Clients
  - Print and Email Volume Client Invoices
  - View Summary of $ Owed by Volume Clients
  - Apply Payments
- Easy Item Sales
- Accounting Reports
  - Reconciliation Report
  - Print Clinic Ledger
- Accounting Tools

Public Client Transactions

After you have begun the checkout process, you may realize that some of your public clients still owe a balance to your clinic that they will need to pay when they pick up their animal. Print a Pickup Balance List for your front desk staff so they know what to collect and from whom. Once you collect from your public clients learn how to apply those payments in Clinic HQ.

Print Pickup Balance List

1. Click on the <Accounting> Icon
2. Click on the blue <Public> link on the left hand main menu
3. Three categories will drop down below the link
4. Select the <Pickup Balance List> category
5. Select the date you wish to print a pickup balance list for (today's date will default)
6. A list of clients and animals is generated, showing how much is still owed for each
7. Click on the blue <PDF> button at the top of the page to create a printer friendly version
8. Adjust your print settings on the left side of the PDF report and click the print button

Apply Payments – Public

1. Click on the <Accounting> Icon
2. Click on the <Public> link on the left hand main menu

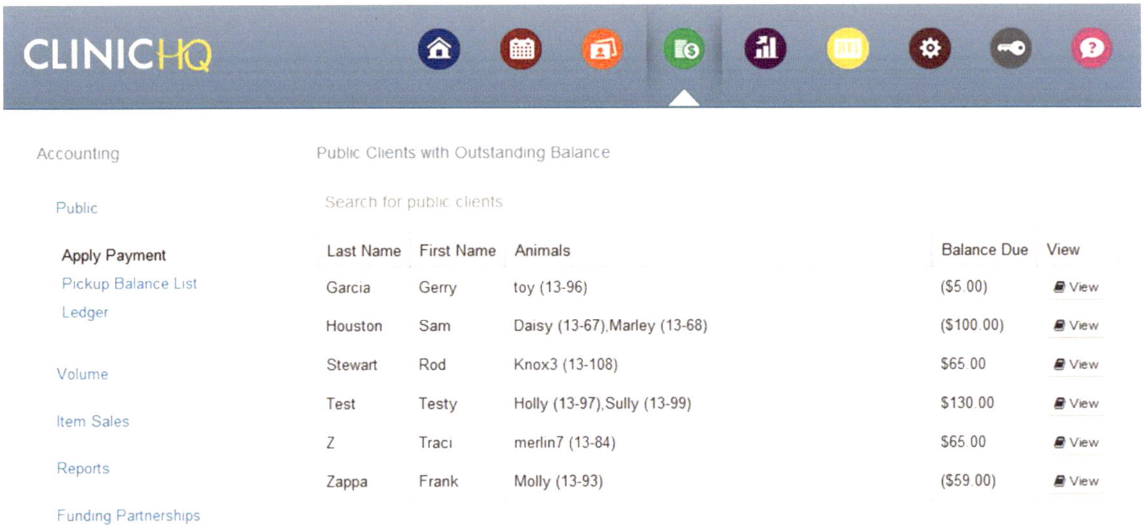

3. Three categories will drop down beneath the link
4. Select <Apply Payment> category
5. A list of public clients with outstanding balances will generate to the right
6. Choose the public client you wish to apply payment to
7. Click the <View> button to the far right of the client's row
8. You will now be taken to the payment screen

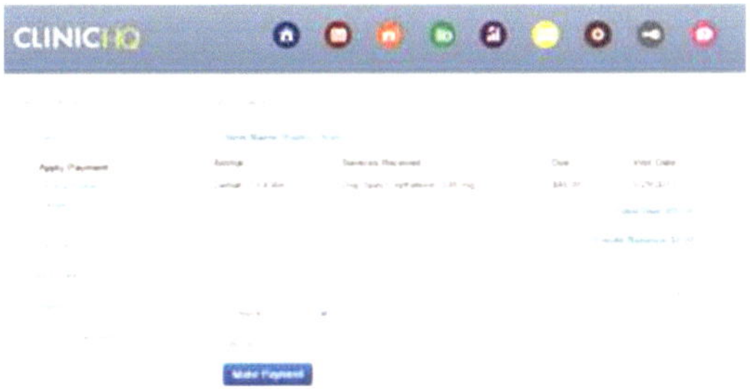

9. Enter the amount of the cash, check, credit card, or secondary subsidy you are applying on this screen

   Note: Only subsidies tied to Flex Funding Partnerships will generate here
10. If paying by check, enter the check number to the right of the amount
11. If paying by credit card, enter the credit card type in the check number field (ex: Visa)
12. If this balance is a write off, enter the amount due in the write off field
13. Click on the blue <Make Payment> button at the bottom to complete

   Note: If you are applying two different forms of payment to one client, you will need to apply each payment separately. They will then appear as two separate line items on your Reconciliation Report.

Volume Client Transactions

Due to the fact that your volume clients will be billed after the fact, you will need a way to keep track of who owes what to your clinic. We will show you how to view a summary of what each volume client owes, print and e-mail invoices, bill your volume clients, and apply their payments once you receive them. Let's get started!

Bill Volume Clients

1. Click on the <Accounting> Icon
2. Click on blue <Volume> link on the left hand main menu
3. Four categories will drop down under the link
4. Choose the <Bill> category
5. All currently unbilled clients will now generate
6. To bill only one client, check the box in their row
7. To bill everyone on this list, check the <Bill &Mail> box at the top of the grid
8. A bill will now be sent to your volume client's e-mail address and it will disappear from this list of unbilled clients

Print and Email Volume Client Invoices

1. Click on the <Accounting> Icon
2. Click on the blue <Volume> link on the left hand main menu
3. Four categories will drop down under the link
4. Choose the <Invoices> category
5. A list will then generate of the most recent invoices for each volume client
6. Click on each blue invoice number to generate each invoice
7. Scroll to the bottom of the invoice to view invoice total
8. Click on either <e-mail> or <print> buttons at the bottom of the page

Note: You can manually enter an e-mail address to send the invoice to, or if you simply click the e-mail button, it will automatically send to the e-mail on file for that client.

View Summary of $ Owed by Volume Clients

1. Click on <Accounting> Icon
2. Click on the blue <Volume> link on the left hand main menu
3. Four categories will drop down under the link
4. Select the <Summary> category
5. This will generate a list of all of your volume clients, their current credit balances, and the total amount that they currently owe your clinic
6. Click on the $ amount in blue to view individual volume client invoices
7. You will now see the breakdown by date and invoice number for all unpaid invoices
8. Click on each blue invoice link to view that invoice
9. You can apply payments from this page as well. We will go over how to perform this function in more detail later in this chapter.

Apply Payments – Volume

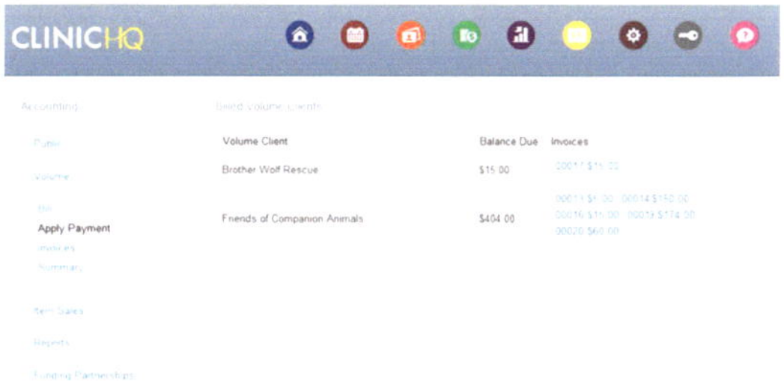

1. Click on the <Accounting> Icon
2. Select <Volume> link from the left hand main menu
3. Four categories will appear below the link
4. Select the blue < Apply Payment> category
5. A list of billed volume clients will generate to the right

6. The total amount owed and links to each individual invoice can be accessed here
7. Click on the blue link for the invoice you would like to apply payment to

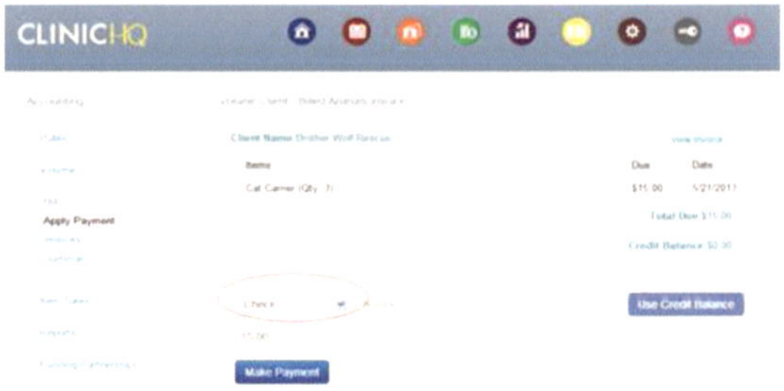

8. From this next screen choose cash, check, or credit card from the drop down menu
9. Enter the amount of the cash, check, or credit card and a check number if applicable
   Note: For credit card payments enter the type of credit card into the check number field.
10. Click the blue <Make Payment> button to save Note: You can click the <Use Credit Balance> button, if you wish to clear an invoice using the client's credits for overpayment etc.

Easy Item Sales

Process easy payments for items you sell specific to your clinic. They do not need to be connected to an animal record, but it will allow you to track how much revenue you are generating from each item.

1. Click on the <Accounting> Icon
2. Click on the blue <Item Sales> link on the left hand main menu
3. To process a sale click the blue <New Sale> button in the top right corner
4. A new screen will generate listing the items you have for sale at your clinic
5. We will show you how to set up these items in Chapter 7
6. From this screen enter the quantity of each item the client is purchasing
7. Click the check box under the <Sell> column next to the selected items
8. Enter payment type from the drop down menu if sold to public client

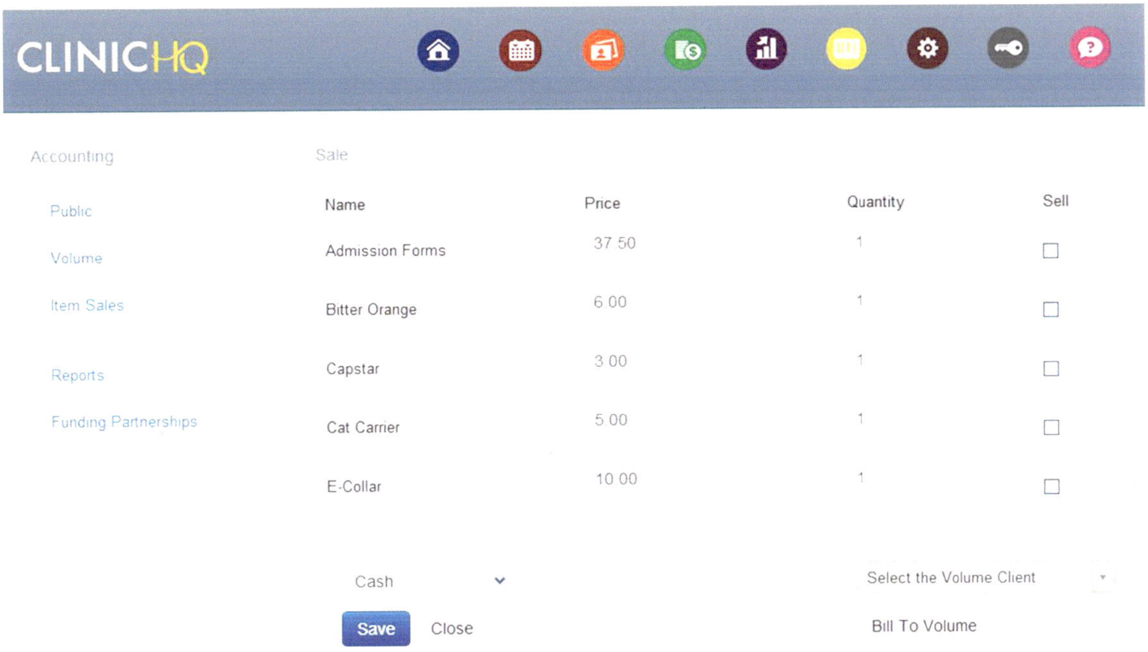

9. Collect the cash or check from the client
10. Click the blue <Save> button to complete the transaction
11. For Volume clients, select their name from the drop down menu on the bottom right
12. Click the <Bill to Volume> button to create an invoice for volume clients

Note: This will not actually bill the volume client. You will still need to go through the billing process for the volume client.

Accounting Reports

To balance your money on hand at the end of every day the Reconciliation Report is invaluable. It will show you exactly how much you took in for the day, and should match up perfectly with your daily deposit. You can also print a Clinic Leger that will show all transactions, including subsidies (discounts), by your specified date range. Let's try it!

Reconciliation Report

1. Click on the <Accounting> Icon
2. Click on the blue <Reports> link on the left hand main menu
3. Two categories will drop down below the link
4. Select the <Reconciliation> category
5. Click the <Search> button
6. This will generate all payments that you have applied for today's date
7. Click on any of the black links at the top of the grid to sort by that category
8. You can click on <Tender>, for example, to separate by cash, check, and credit card receipts.
9. Scroll to the bottom of the screen for your grand total

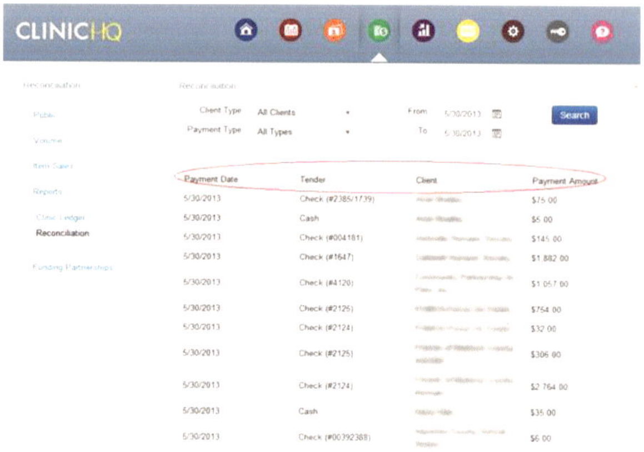

Note: You can narrow your search with the drop down menus at the top of the page

Clinic Ledger

1. Click on the <Accounting> Icon
2. Click on the blue <Reports> link on the left hand main menu
3. Two categories will drop down from the link
4. Select the <Clinic Ledger> category
5. On the screen to the right, you will see two data boxes for date range
6. Input the beginning and end date you wish to view
7. The report will generate on a new page that looks like this

8. Right click on the screen with your mouse and select print option
9. Scroll to the bottom of the page for a grand total

Accounting Tools

Nobody is perfect and sometimes mistakes do happen. But not to worry, because when they do, we've got you covered! Clinic HQ has developed specific tools in our Accounting section to fix some pretty common errors very easily. Here are a couple of scenarios where they can help.

Wrong Subsidy was Applied then Billed to Wrong Volume Client

1. Click on <Accounting> Icon
2. Click on blue <Tools> link from the left hand main menu
3. Click the <Go> button to the right of the first tool <Incorrect Subsidy Applied>

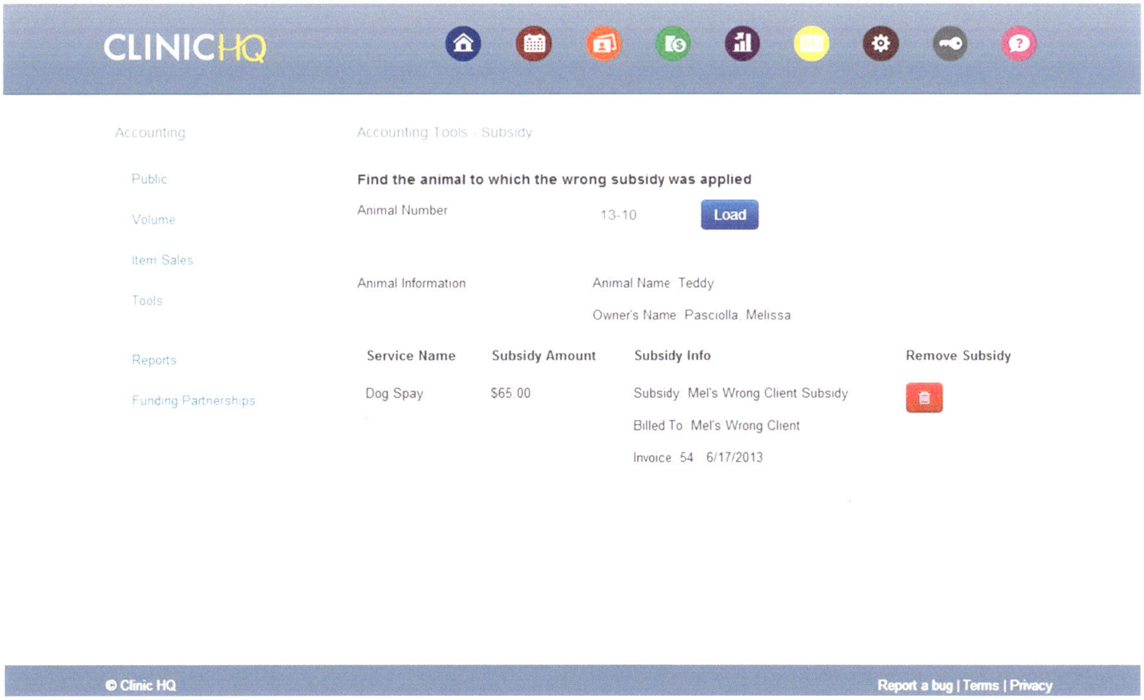

4. Enter the animal ID number that you billed incorrectly
5. Click the blue <Load> button
6. The animal record information you searched for should generate below
7. Click on the red garbage can to remove this incorrect subsidy
8. A <New Subsidy> drop down menu will now generate
9. Select the new subsidy you want to apply
10. Select <Yes> button to remove this animal from the previously billed invoice, and to bill it to the new volume client

Incorrect Payment Applied to an Invoice

1. Click on <Accounting> Icon
2. Click on blue <Tools> link from the left hand main menu
3. Click the <Go> button to the right of the second tool <Incorrect Payment Applied – Invoice>
4. Enter the invoice number you have paid incorrectly
5. Click the <Load> button
6. The payment information for this invoice will generate below
7. Click the red garbage can to remove the incorrect payment
8. Select <Yes> if you are sure you want to delete the payment

Continuous updates will occur with Accounting Tools.
Keep checking in!

Chapter

5

Reports

While you are entering data, Clinic HQ is doing some behind the scenes work for you. It is carefully creating useful reports with your data and tracking all of the metrics that are critical to your clinic. In this chapter we will show you how to utilize the following reports by metric:

- Patient
- Service
- Volume Client
- Geographic
- Partnership
- BONUS Reminder Logs*

Patient Metric Report

This report will allow you to view statistics related to all patients who have come through your clinic within a selected time frame. Break this report down by surgery stats, by animal, or by appointment data. All of this information is available monthly, yearly, or quarterly. Let's take a look!

To View/Print Surgery Statistics

This report will show successful surgery statistics, broken down by type of animal, type of surgery, and death stats.

1. Click on <Reports> Icon
2. The default view is the Patient Metrics page
3. This page also defaults to <Surgeries> view
4. From the drop down fields at the top of the page select the year and quarter you would like to view.

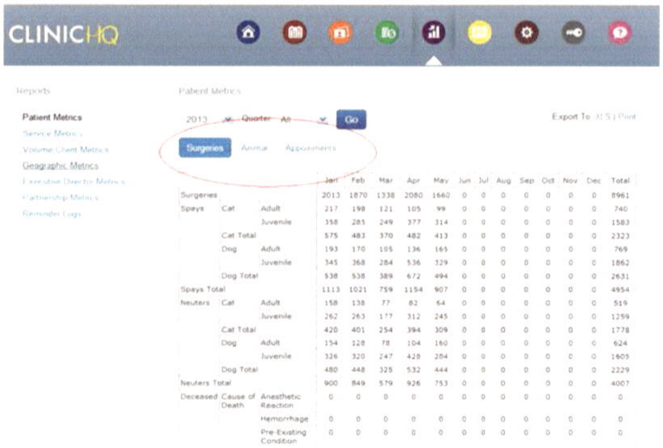

5. Click on the blue <Go> button to generate report
6. Export this report to Excel or a printable view by clicking the desired link in the upper right hand corner of the patient metrics screen

To View/Print Animal Statistics

This report will give a total number of animals that have visited the clinic, whether or not their surgeries were successful and a detailed breakdown of those visiting animals.

1. Click on <Reports> Icon
2. The default view is the Patient Metrics page
3. Click on blue <Animal> Button at the top of the page
4. From the drop down fields at the top of the page select the year and quarter you would like to view
5. Click on the blue <Go> button to generate report
6. Export this report to Excel or a printable view by clicking on the desired links in the upper right hand corner of the patient metrics screen

To View/Print Appointment Statistics

This report reflects the number of appointments processed at your clinic in the past, present, and future.

1. Click on <Reports> Icon
2. The default view is the Patient Metrics page

3. Click on blue <Appointment> Button at the top of the page
4. From the drop down fields at the top of the page select the year and quarter you would like to view
5. Click on the blue <Go> button to generate report
6. Export this report to Excel or a printable view by clicking on the desired links in the upper right hand corner of the patient metrics screen

Service Metric Report

View all metrics related to the services and products you offer at your clinic. This includes all item sales, surgeries, vaccines, and any additional products you may sell. This list of services and products is tailored to your specific clinic, in the Settings section of Clinic HQ. We will show you how to set up your products and services in **Chapter 7**.

To View/Print Service Data

1. Click on <Reports> Icon
2. Click on the blue <Service Metrics> link on the left hand main menu
3. From the drop down fields at the top of the page select the year and quarter you would like to view
4. Click on the blue <Go> button to generate report
5. Export this report to Excel or a printable view by clicking on the desired link in the upper right hand corner of the reports screen

Volume Client Metric Report

Your volume clients are a very large part of the business that you do at your clinic. The Volume Client Metric Report gives you a breakdown of how many animals per volume client you have seen by the month, quarter, and year to date. It also gives you an option to view what percentage of total business each volume client is giving you. Plus, it provides a detailed report of what type of animals your volume clients are bringing in and how many of each. (Ex: sheltered, fostered, owned, feral, etc.) Remember, all of this data will be specific to your clinic.

View/ Print Volume Client Numbers

1. Click on <Reports> Icon
2. Click on the blue <Volume Client Metrics> link on the left hand main menu
3. Screen will default to <Numbers> tab
4. From the drop down fields at the top of the page select the year and quarter you would like to view
5. Click on the blue <Go> button to generate report
6. Export this report to Excel or a printable view by clicking on the desired link in the upper right hand corner of the reports screen

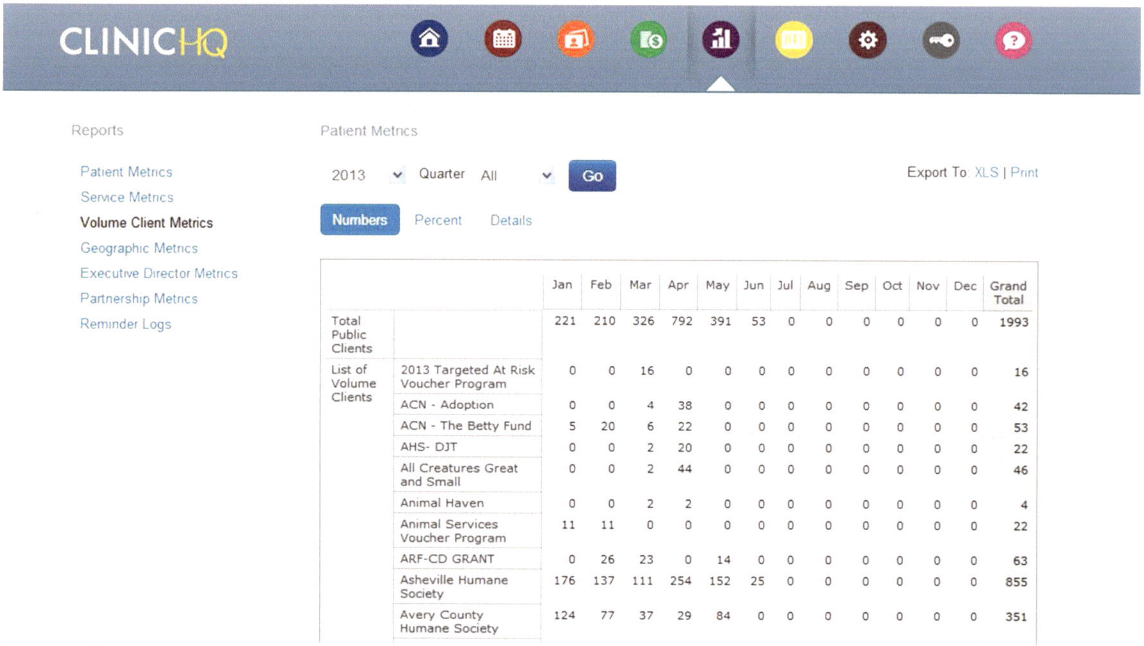

		Jan	Feb	Mar	Apr	May	Jun	Jul	Aug	Sep	Oct	Nov	Dec	Grand Total
Total Public Clients		221	210	326	792	391	53	0	0	0	0	0	0	1993
List of Volume Clients	2013 Targeted At Risk Voucher Program	0	0	16	0	0	0	0	0	0	0	0	0	16
	ACN - Adoption	0	0	4	38	0	0	0	0	0	0	0	0	42
	ACN - The Betty Fund	5	20	6	22	0	0	0	0	0	0	0	0	53
	AHS- DJT	0	0	2	20	0	0	0	0	0	0	0	0	22
	All Creatures Great and Small	0	0	2	44	0	0	0	0	0	0	0	0	46
	Animal Haven	0	0	2	2	0	0	0	0	0	0	0	0	4
	Animal Services Voucher Program	11	11	0	0	0	0	0	0	0	0	0	0	22
	ARF-CD GRANT	0	26	23	0	14	0	0	0	0	0	0	0	63
	Asheville Humane Society	176	137	111	254	152	25	0	0	0	0	0	0	855
	Avery County Humane Society	124	77	37	29	84	0	0	0	0	0	0	0	351

View/ Print Volume Client Percentages

1. Click on <Reports> Icon
2. Click on the blue <Volume Client Metrics> link on the left hand main menu
3. Click on the blue <Percent> button to the right of the <Numbers> button
4. From the drop down fields at the top of the page select the year and quarter you would like to view
5. Click on the blue <Go> button to generate report
6. Export this report to Excel or a printable view by clicking on the desired link in the upper right hand corner of the reports screen

View/ Print Volume Client Details

1. Click on <Reports> Icon
2. Click on the blue <Volume Client Metrics> link on the left hand main menu
3. Click on the blue <Details> button to the right of the <Percent> button
4. From the drop down fields at the top of the page select the year and quarter you would like to view
5. Click on the blue <Go> button to generate report
6. Export this report to Excel or a printable view by clicking on the desired link in the upper right hand corner of the reports screen

Geographic Metrics

This may be the most exciting report in Clinic HQ. Your data entry will actually serve the entire spay and neuter community through this mapping software! Every time you enter a client's address, it is transformed into a small dot on this map. This will eventually allow you and all other Clinic HQ clinics to see where animals are and are not being spayed and neutered, and where there is a need for new clinics! Here's how to navigate the map!

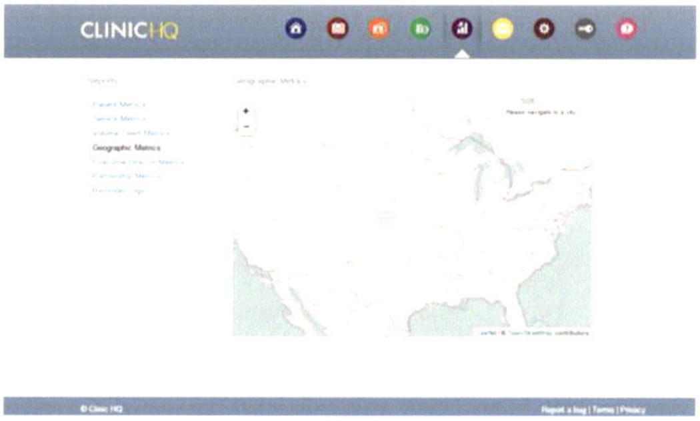

1. Click on <Reports> Icon
2. Click on the blue <Geographic Metrics> link on the left hand main menu
3. You will now see a map of the U.S.
4. Hover your mouse (looks like a hand) over the map and double click to zoom
5. Zoom all the way in to the city you wish to view right down to individual streets!

Partnership Metric Report

You have built incredible partnerships with your local shelters and rescue groups. This report is a breakdown of all of your volume clients and the number and types of services you are supplying for them. You can view this report quarterly or track by month for any selected year!

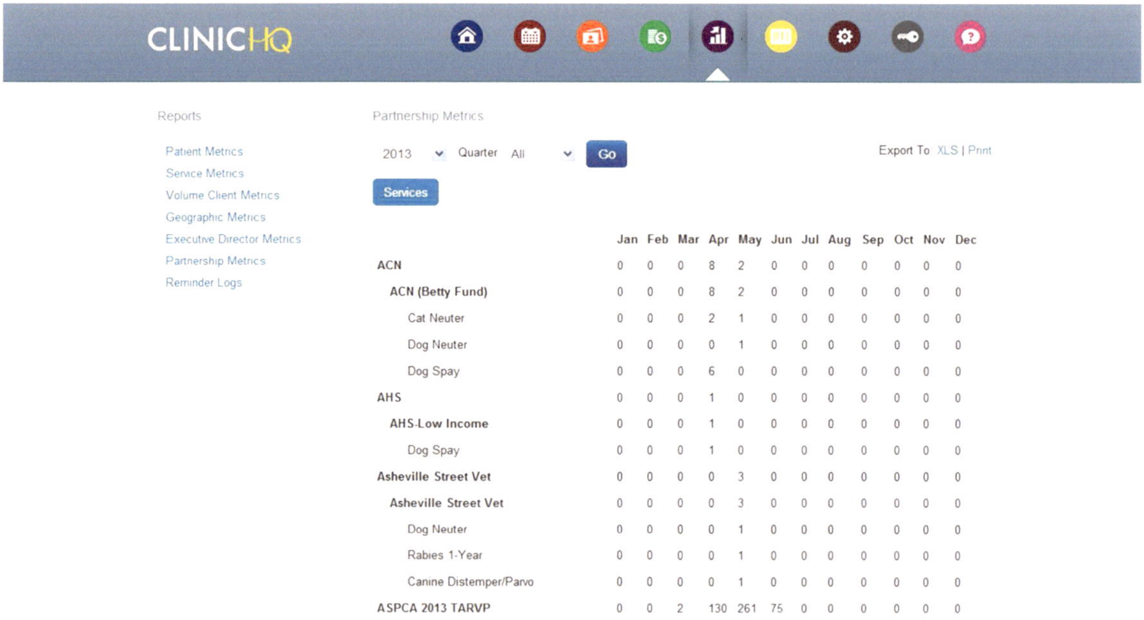

	Jan	Feb	Mar	Apr	May	Jun	Jul	Aug	Sep	Oct	Nov	Dec
ACN	0	0	0	8	2	0	0	0	0	0	0	0
ACN (Betty Fund)	0	0	0	8	2	0	0	0	0	0	0	0
Cat Neuter	0	0	0	2	1	0	0	0	0	0	0	0
Dog Neuter	0	0	0	0	1	0	0	0	0	0	0	0
Dog Spay	0	0	0	6	0	0	0	0	0	0	0	0
AHS	0	0	0	1	0	0	0	0	0	0	0	0
AHS-Low Income	0	0	0	1	0	0	0	0	0	0	0	0
Dog Spay	0	0	0	1	0	0	0	0	0	0	0	0
Asheville Street Vet	0	0	0	0	3	0	0	0	0	0	0	0
Asheville Street Vet	0	0	0	0	3	0	0	0	0	0	0	0
Dog Neuter	0	0	0	0	1	0	0	0	0	0	0	0
Rabies 1-Year	0	0	0	0	1	0	0	0	0	0	0	0
Canine Distemper/Parvo	0	0	0	0	1	0	0	0	0	0	0	0
ASPCA 2013 TARVP	0	0	2	130	261	75	0	0	0	0	0	0

1. Click on <Reports> Icon
2. Click on blue <Partnership Metric> link on the left hand main menu
3. Select the year and quarter you wish to view from the drop down menus
4. Click <Go> Button to generate report
5. Export this report to Excel or a printable view by clicking on the desired link in the upper right hand corner of the reports screen

*Bonus – Reminder Logs

This condensed report will help you keep track of all of the reminders you have sent out to your clients. We will show you how to create reminders in Chapter 7. It will display what type of reminder you have sent, the date, and the client's information. Just think of it as a little reminder for you about your reminders! Let's take a look.

1. Click on the <Reports> Icon
2. Click on the blue < Reminder Logs> link on the left hand main menu
3. The most recent reminders will automatically populate on your screen
4. Click on the <Details> link to the right of the client's name to view all information about the call, e-mail, or text that was sent to the client.
5. To view older reminders scroll to the bottom of the page, and select <Older> link

Chapter

6

Settings

When you sign up for your Clinic HQ software, our staff will do a one hour set up with key members of your admin staff. We will help you tailor your system to your specific clinic during this session. This chapter will review that setup process, so if you need to adjust anything in the future, you can refer to this manual. The Settings section of Clinic HQ is the foundation for all other functions in the program, and we're going to show you how to use it!

- Set up Clinic Profile
- Add New Species (dog & cat default)
- Manage Services and Products Offered
  - Surgery Types
  - Vaccines
  - Additional Services & Products
  - Items for Sale
- Capacity Management
- Create & Manage Funding Partnerships
- Create & Manage Subsidies
- Manage Vet Profiles
- Manage Clinic HQ User Profiles
- Set Rabies Tag Allotments
- Create Client Reminders

Set up Clinic Profile

If you ever have any need to update your clinic's information (ex: address, phone number, logo, etc.) this is where you will do it. There are five tabs under this section that we will explore:

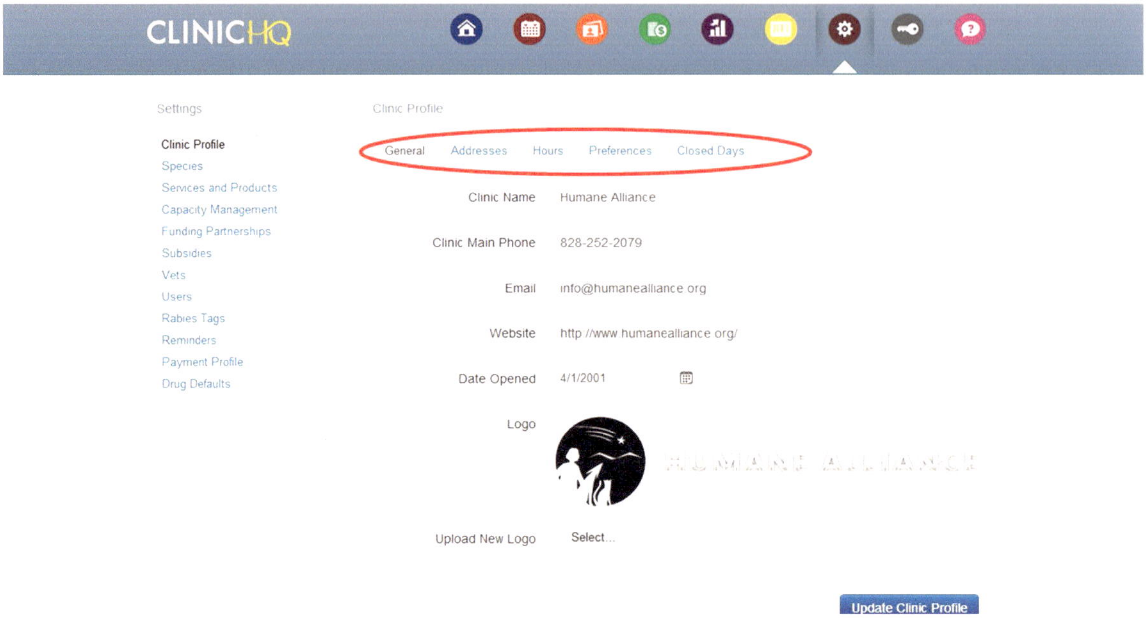

- General
- Addresses
- Hours
- Preferences
- Closed Days

General

1. Click <Settings> Icon
2. Click on blue <Clinic Profile> link on the left hand main menu
3. The screen will default to the <General> tab

4. Enter your clinic's information into the appropriate fields
5. To upload your logo, click on the <Select> button
6. This will pull up all of your computer files
7. Select your logo and click <Open> to upload the logo to Clinic HQ

   Note: The size of your logo should not exceed 300 x 60
8. To save your changes, click blue <Update Clinic Profile> button

Addresses

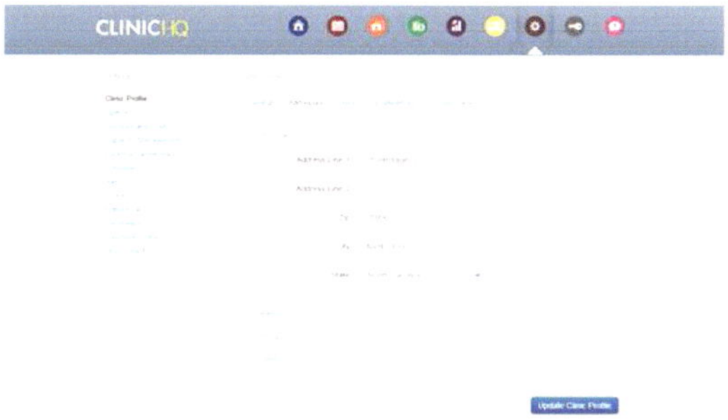

1. Click on <Settings> Icon
2. Click on blue <Clinic Profile> link on the left hand main menu
3. Click on the blue <Addresses> tab at the top of the screen
4. Enter your clinic's physical address
5. Click on the blue <Mailing> link
6. Enter your clinic's mailing address (where you receive your mail, can be a P.O. box)
7. If it is the same as your physical address click the check box
8. Click on the blue <Billing> link
9. Enter your clinic's billing address (where you receive your bills from vendors)
10. If it is the same as your physical address click the check box
11. Click the blue <Remit> link
12. Enter your clinic's remit address (where your client's should send payments to you)
13. If it is the same as your physical address click the check box
14. Click the blue <Update Clinic Profile> button to save your changes

Hours

1. Click on <Settings> Icon
2. Click on blue <Clinic Profile> link on the left hand main menu
3. Click on the <Hours> tab at the top of the screen
4. Set your clinic opening and closing hours for each day of the week.
5. To set a day as closed, click on the check boxes under the <Closed Day> column
6. Click the <Update Clinic Profile> button to save your changes

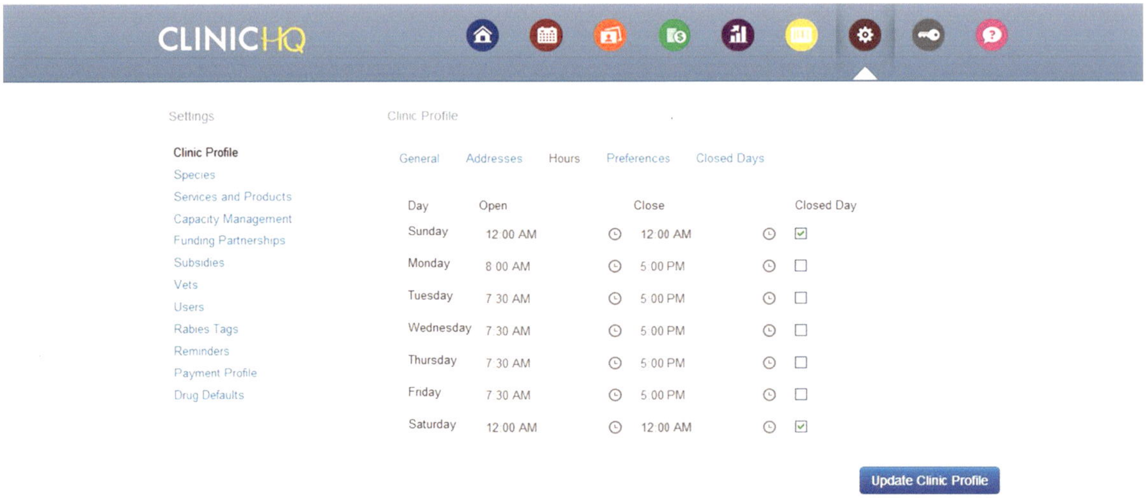

Preferences

1. Click on <Settings> Icon
2. Click on blue <Clinic Profile> link on the left hand main menu
3. Click on the <Preferences> tab at the top of the page
4. Check the <Does this clinic accept credit cards> box (optional)
5. There will also be two Invoice CC email fields. Enter two email addresses that

you wish to have copied when invoices are sent from Clinic HQ. (optional)

6. Click <Update Clinic Profile> button to save your changes

Closed Days

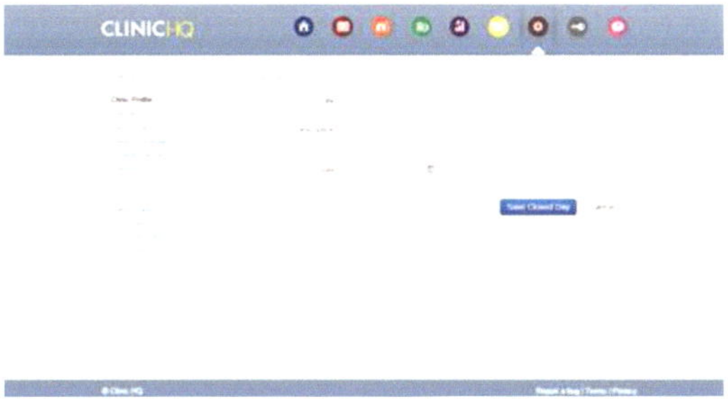

1. Click on <Settings> Icon
2. Click on blue <Clinic Profile> link on the left hand main menu
3. Click on the <Closed Days> tab at the top of the screen
4. We have listed general holidays that you may be closed on this page
5. If your clinic does not close on one of these day, click the <delete> button to re move it
6. To add a closed day click on the <+Create Closed Day> link at the top of the grid
7. Title your closed day, enter its description, and select the date.
8. Click <Save Closed Day> button to generate your new closed day

Add New Species

Clinic HQ automatically defaults to dogs and cats as the two species you will be performing surgeries on at your clinic. If your clinic sees other types of animals, this is where you can add them into the system.

1. Click on <Settings> Icon
2. Click on the blue <Species> link on the left hand main menu
3. You will see a grid with cat and dog listed as your two species of animal
4. Click on the blue <Create Species> link in the upper right hand corner of the grid

5. Enter the type of animal under <Title> and any additional description beneath it
6. Click the <Save> button to add this new species

Manage Services and Products Offered

Throughout Clinic HQ you will add on services and products to client records and bills, sell individual items to walk in clients, and track all of the above in valuable reports. This is where you will set up all of those services and products that are specific to your clinic, and their respective pricing. We will break this section down into the following categories:

- Surgery Types
- Vaccines
- Additional Services & Products
- Items for Sale

Surgery Types

1. Click on <Settings> Icon
2. Click on the blue <Services and Products> link from the left hand main menu
3. Screen will default to <Surgery Types> Tab
4. The Surgeries you have told us that you do at your clinic will now generate.
5. Change your Public and Volume costs here.
6. Make sure the check boxes are checked if you currently perform each type of surgery. This will make them active in the system. Uncheck any surgeries you do not perform.
7. Click the <Save> button to update your changes

There are only 4 basic types of surgery in Clinic HQ:
Dog Spay/Dog Neuter
Cat Spay/Cat Neuter
If you charge additional fees for larger dogs, for example, we would add that extra fee in as an additional service or product for your clinic.

Vaccines

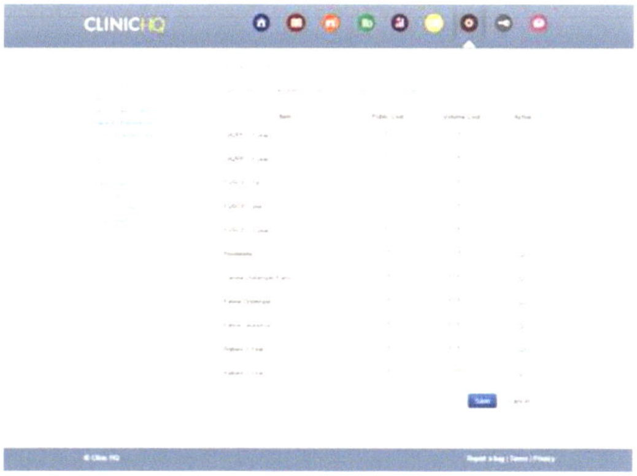

1. Click on the <Settings> Icon
2. Click on the blue <Services and Products> link from the left hand main menu
3. Select the <Vaccines> tab to the right of the default <Surgery Types> tab
4. A grid with pre-set vaccines your clinic may use will generate
5. If your clinic uses the vaccine, click on the check box to activate it
6. You can edit the pricing for public and volume clients here
7. Click the <Save> button to update your changes

Additional Services & Products

1. Click on the <Settings> Icon
2. Click on the blue <Services and Products> link from the left hand main menu
3. Select the <Services> tab to the right of the <Vaccines> tab at the top of the page

4. A grid of all of the possible services your clinic may offer will generate
5. For each service your clinic offers, click on the check boxes to activate them
6. You can edit pricing for public and volume clients here as well
7. Click the <Save> button to update your changes
8. Click on the <Products> tab to the right of the <Services> tab
9. Repeat the above process to set your pricing and activate the <Products> your clinic offers

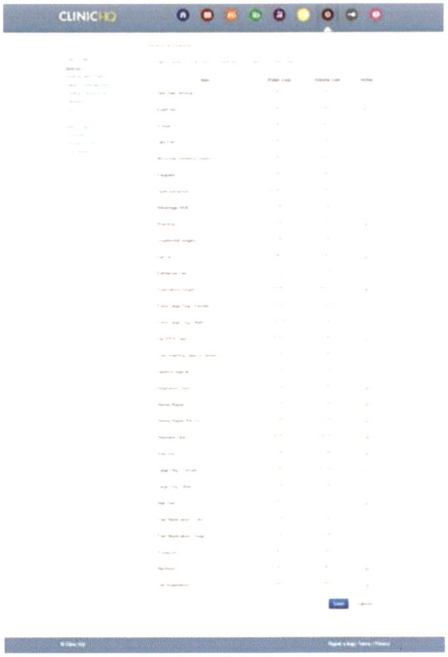

Item Sales

1. Click on the <Settings> Icon

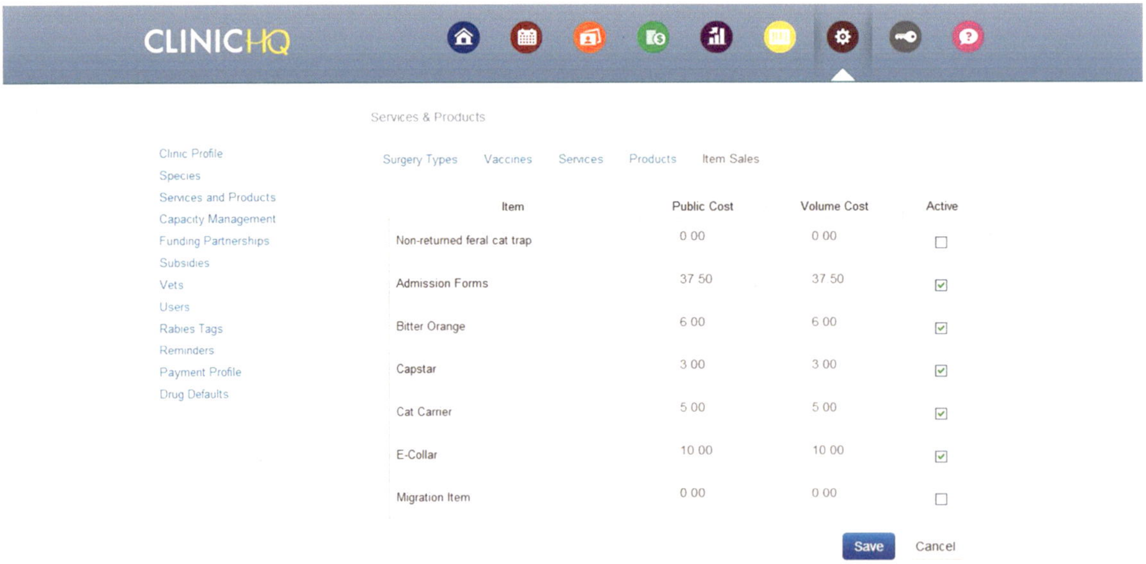

2. Click on the blue <Services and Products> link from the left hand main menu
3. Select the <Item Sales> tab to the right of the <Products> tab at the top of the page
4. A list of all of the items you will sell, that do not need to be attached to an animal record, will generate here
5. For each item your clinic sells, click on the check boxes to activate them
6. Edit the prices for volume and public clients here and don't forget to <SAVE>

Capacity Management

One of the most crucial elements to running a smooth clinic operation is properly setting your daily capacity. How many of each type of surgery can your vet staff complete in a day's time? The information that you enter in this section will then appear on your Calendar, so that those making appointments for your clinic will know when you are nearing, or have met your capacity for any given day. The information that you enter here will be very specific to your individual clinic. Let's show you how!

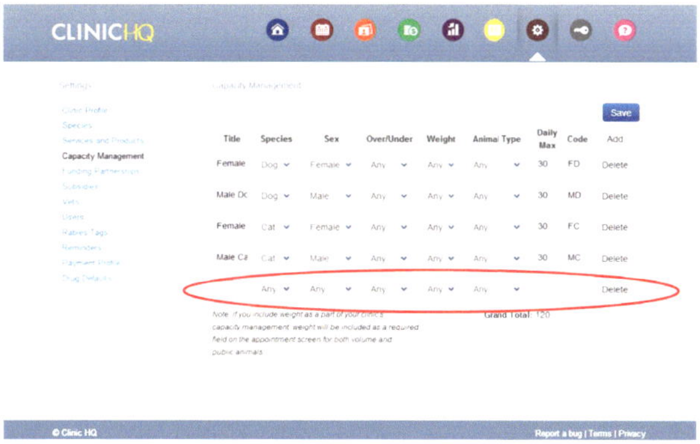

1. Click on the <Settings> Icon
2. Click on the blue <Capacity Management> link from the left hand main menu
3. To add your first appointment category click the <Add> button at the top right hand corner of the generated grid
4. Work from left to right to fill in the fields
5. Title will be for example: Female Dog
6. Species would be: Dog

7. Sex: Female

Title	Species	Sex	Over/Under	Weight	Animal Type	Daily Max	Code	Add
FD	Dog	Female	Any	Any	Any	30	FD	Delete

8. If your clinic classifies surgeries based on weight enter this information, if they do not leave as <Any>
9. If your clinic classifies surgeries based on animal type (ex: owned, sheltered, feral, etc.) enter this information, if they do not leave as <Any>
10. Enter Daily Maximum for this type of surgery Note: After you have entered all of your daily maximums for each type of animal surgery, the total number of surgeries should be what your clinic vets can handle in a day.
11. Enter calendar code for this type of surgery (ex: FD for Female Dog) This can be a max of three letters

Your clinic can add as many types of surgeries as you wish to track for your vets. You may have small, medium, and large male dogs; making a total of 3 tiles just for your male dog surgeries on your calendar. Basically, the sky is the limit when it comes to Capacity Management in Clinic HQ!

12. Click the <Save> button to update your new classification of appointment
13. Repeat this process as many times as necessary to add every classification of animal surgery your clinic needs to track

Create and Manage Funding Partnerships

There are three possible types of Funding Partnerships that can be set up in Clinic HQ. The first type is set up so that an organization that offers the public discounts on services at your clinic is invoiced and billed by your clinic for those services. The second type exists when donations of large sums of money create a pot that can be deducted from when vouchers are presented to your clinic. The third type will be a flexible pot of money that can be applied to public client invoices to cover any additional balance owed. This type of funding partnership is perfect to connect to donation jars etc. We are now going to show you how to set up and edit each type of Funding Partnership.

- Invoiced Funding Partnership
- Prepaid Funding Partnership
- Flexible Funding Partnership

When to use each type of Funding Partnership?

Invoiced: Perfect for when one of your Volume Clients, like a local shelter, sets up a voucher program for public clients to use. When the public clients turn in these vouchers for free or discounted services at your clinic, you would then bill the Volume Client for those services.

Prepaid: Any time your clinic receives a grant or sum of money to be drawn down from, for public or volume services, this type of Funding Partnership should be set up. It can also often used in conjunction with voucher programs. Whenever you use a discount tied to this Funding Partnership, that amount will be deducted from that pot of money, and Clinic HQ will track that deduction so you always know your current balance.

Flexible: This type of Funding Partnership is perfect for donation jars and other small pots of money that can be used as secondary subsidies to cover remaining balances for clients that may not be able to pay their bill.

Create Invoiced Funding Partnership

1. Click on <Settings> Icon
2. Click on blue <Funding Partnerships> link from the left hand main menu
3. Click on <+Create Grant> link in the upper right hand corner of the generated grid
4. Select <Invoiced> from grant type drop down menu

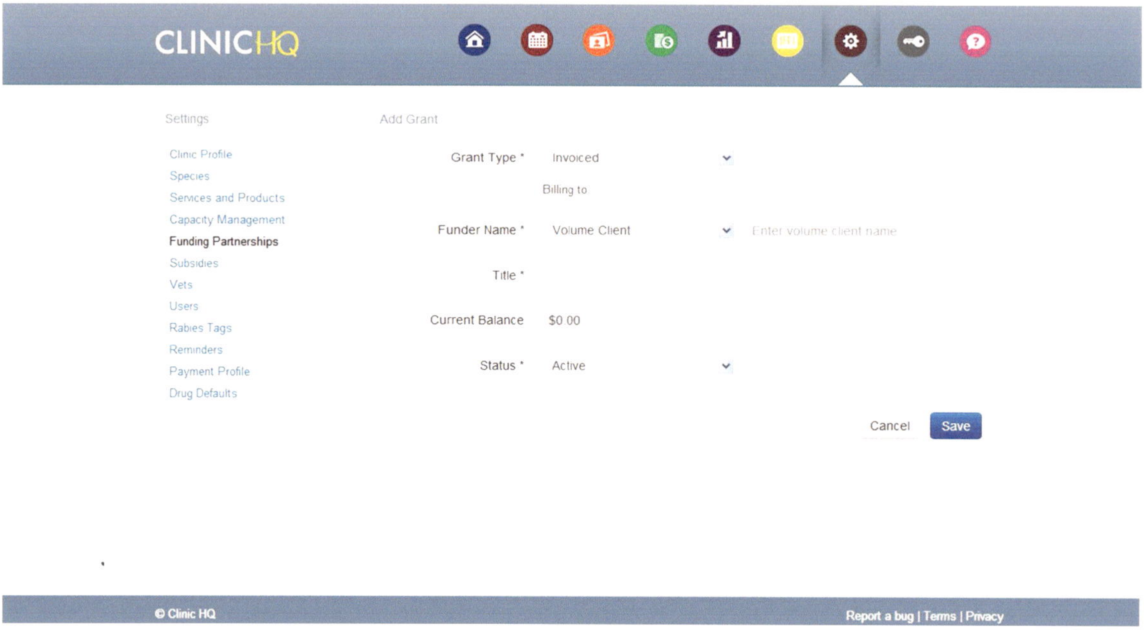

5. Select <Volume Client> from funder name drop down menu
6. A new text box will appear to the right of the <Volume Client> selection
7. Enter a previously created Volume Client Note: The Volume Client you enter has to have been created previously, or you will not be able to create invoices for them.
8. Enter the name of this new Funding Partnership in the <Title> field
9. Leave the current balance at $0

10. Make sure <Status> is set to <Active>
11. Click <Save> button to create your new Funding Partnership

Create Prepaid Funding Partnership

1. Click on <Settings> Icon
2. Click on blue <Funding Partnerships> link from the left hand main menu
3. Click on <+Create Grant> link in the upper right hand corner of the generated grid
4. Select <Prepaid> from grant type drop down menu
5. Select <New> from funder name drop down menu
6. Enter <Funder Name>
7. Enter the name of this Funding Partnership in the <Title> field

Note: It can be the same as the <Funder Name>

8. Leave the current balance at $0 for now

   Note: We will show you how to change this balance when we edit the funding partnership.
9. Make sure <Status> is set to <Active>
10. Click <Save> button to create your new Funding Partnership

Create Flexible Funding Partnership

1. Click on <Settings> Icon
2. Click on blue <Funding Partnerships> link from the left hand main menu
3. Click on <+Create Grant> link in the upper right hand corner of the generated grid
4. Select <Flex> from grant type drop down menu

5. Select <New> from <Name of Funder> drop down menu
6. Enter <Funder Name> to the right of the drop down
7. Enter the name of this Funding Partnership in the <Title> field Note: It can be the same as the <Funder Name>
8. Leave the current balance at $0 for now
   Note: We will show you how to change this balance when we edit the funding partnership.
9. If this new Funding Partnership is associated with any of the charities listed in the <Associate With> drop down menu, select here. Note: This is very important, because these charities have requested detailed reports that this option will now allow Clinic HQ to generate.
10. Check the donation box, if this fund was created by donations
11. Make sure <Status> is set to <Active> and then click <Save>

Any subsidy tied to this type of funding partnership can also be used as a secondary subsidy to cover remaining balances for public clients!

However, when you use these subsidies as secondary subsidies, to cover remaining balances, they will not count toward your Funding Partnership Metric Report.

Edit Funding Partnerships

1. Click on <Settings> Icon
2. Click on blue <Funding Partnerships> link from the left hand main menu
3. Your list of Funding Partnerships will generate

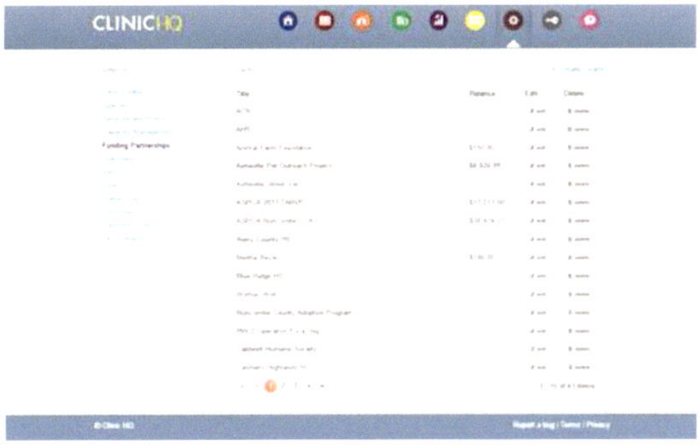

4. There will be a – in the balance column for invoiced funding partnerships
5. There will be the $ amount of the current balance for prepaid funding partnerships
6. Click the <Edit> button next to the FP you wish to change
7. To add money to a pot for a pre-paid or flex FP simply input the amount you would like to add in the <Amount to add/subtract> field

   Note: This is where you will enter your beginning balance for your Funding Partnership, once it is created!
8. You must then enter a description of the funds you are adding. This can be anything you wish, but should give you valuable information about the addition.
9. Click the <Save> button to update your current balance for the FP
10. You can edit any of the information on this page
11. Don't forget to <Save> your changes
12. To delete a FP, simply click the <Delete> button to the right of the <Edit> button on your list of Funding Partnerships

Create and Manage Subsidies

Now that you have created a foundation with your Funding Partnerships, you will be able to add subsidies (discount programs) that will be connected to your Funding Partnerships. These subsidies will then be available for you to apply to client checkouts, reducing or altogether removing the cost of the services for that animal.

Let's dig in!

Multiple subsidies can be set up for each Funding Partnership.

So, if the ASPCA gives you a grant, you can have a subsidy for just cats in a certain zip code and one for female dogs in a certain county that are both pulling from the same pot of money!

Create New Subsidy

1. Click on <Settings> Icon
2. Click on blue <Subsidies> link from the left hand main menu
3. A list of previously created subsidies will generate
4. Click on the blue <+Create Subsidy> link in the upper right hand corner of the grid

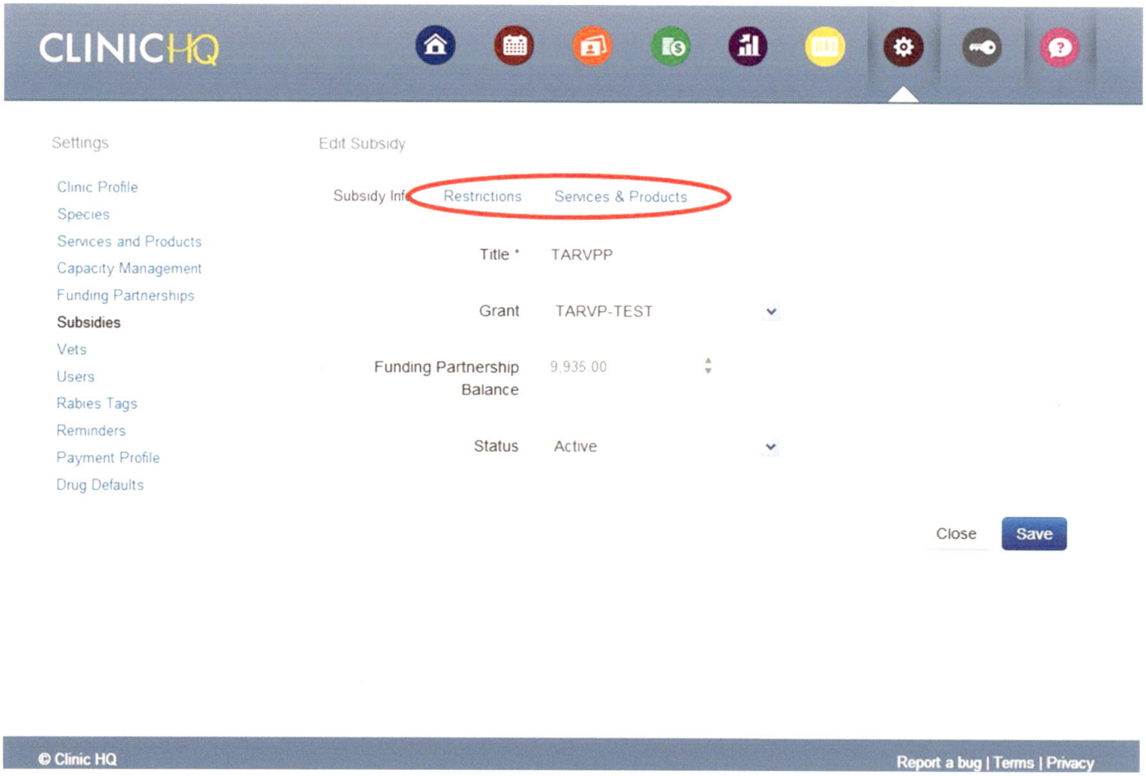

5. Enter the name of this subsidy in the <Title> field
6. Choose Funding Partnership that this subsidy will be tied to from <Grant> drop down
7. Make sure status is <Active>
8. Click <Save> button
9. This will then bring up two additional tabs
10. Click on the <Restrictions> tab
11. Enter any restrictions for this subsidy. For example: If this subsidy is only valid for public clients within a certain county or zip code, enter that information here
12. If there are no restrictions to use this subsidy, click the check box
13. Click the <Save> button to update this page
14. Click on the <Services and Products> tab
15. A list of all of the services and products that you offer at your clinic will generate
16. Click the <+> next to all of the services and products that this subsidy will apply to

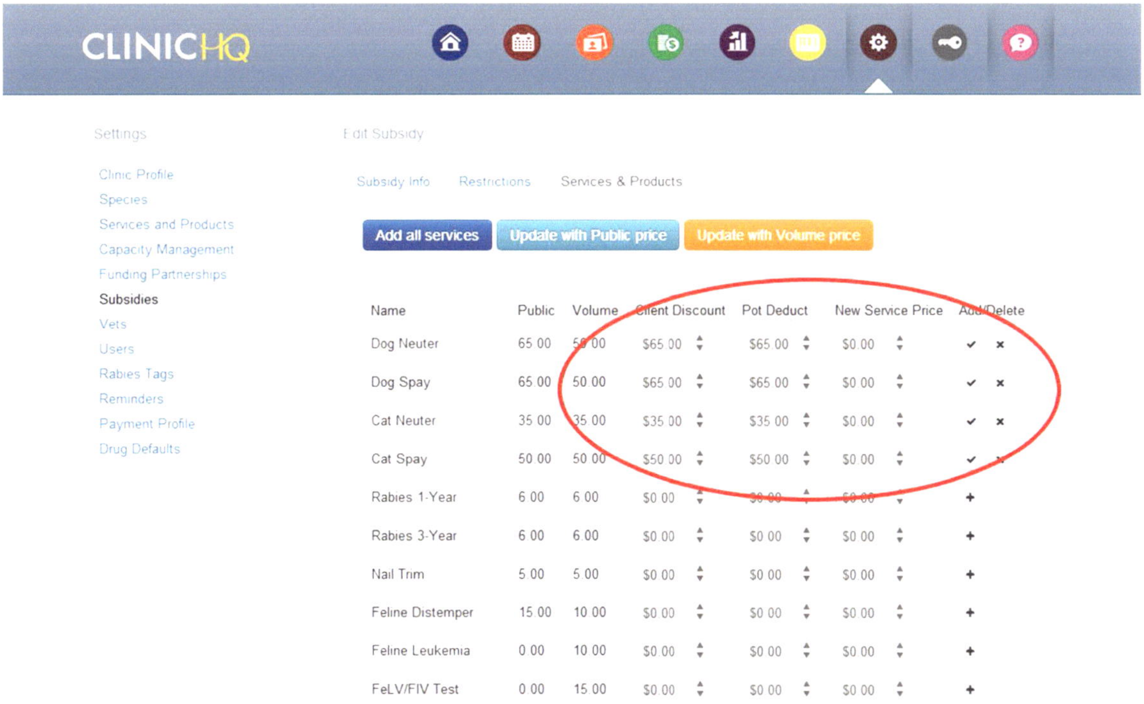

17. Enter the <Client Discount> price when they use this subsidy
18. Enter the <Pot Deduct> or <Bill Volume Client> amount

    Note: Should match <Client Discount> price if covering the entire service or product
19. Click the <Save> button at the bottom of the page to update changes

Edit Subsidies

1. Click on <Settings> Icon
2. Click on blue <Subsidies> link from the left hand main menu
3. A list of all of your currently created subsidies will generate
4. Choose the subsidy you wish to edit
5. Click on the <Edit> button to the right of the subsidy
6. The same three tabs you used to set up this subsidy will reappear
7. Edit the sections you need to change, and don't forget to save each tab
8. To delete a subsidy, simply click the <Delete> button to the right of the <Edit> button on the main subsidy screen.

Manage Vet Profiles

In this section we will teach you how to create a vet profile for each of your vets on staff, manage their schedules, and upload their digital signatures for rabies certificates. Let's try it!

Create Vet Profile

1. Click on the <Settings> Icon
2. Click on the blue <Vets> link from the left hand main menu
3. Click on the blue <+Create Vet> link in the upper right hand corner of the generated grid

4. Choose vet type from the drop down menu

   Note: Humane Alliance has 7 vets who perform different functions each day. If you only have a surgery vet, select <Clinic> from the drop down menu

5. Fill in the rest of the open fields on this page
6. To upload a signature, click the <Select> button at the bottom of the screen.
7. Choose the vet signature file in your computer and click <Open>

   Note: This signature will now automatically be added to any rabies certificate associated with this vet!

8. Click the <Save> button at the bottom of the screen to create vet profile
9. To edit this profile, click on <Edit> button on the main <Vets> screen next to the vet's name

Create Vet Schedule

1. Click on <Settings> Icon
2. Click on blue <Vets> link from the left hand main menu
3. Next to the vet profile of your choosing, click on <+Schedule> button
4. The default tab is the base schedule
5. Enter when this schedule will start and end
6. Click to check the boxes for the days of the week that his vet will work
7. Select when this schedule will repeat
8. Click <Save>
9. Click on <Exclusions> tab at the top of the page

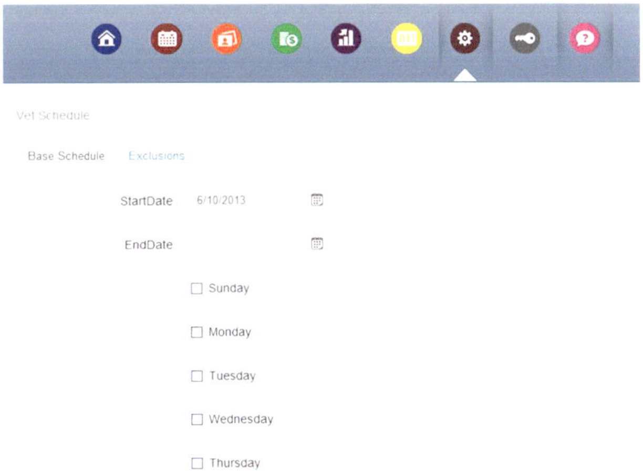

10. Click on <+Add New Record> button
11. Enter start and end date of any vacations or personal days off this vet has scheduled
12. Click <Update> button to the right of the record to save

Manage Clinic HQ User Profiles

Every individual at your clinic that will use Clinic HQ will have their own user profile. It will contain their Clinic HQ log in information and their user access level. We will show you how to create new users when you add to your staff, and how to edit what they will and will not have access to in the system. This will allow even your volunteers to use Clinic HQ!

Create User Roles

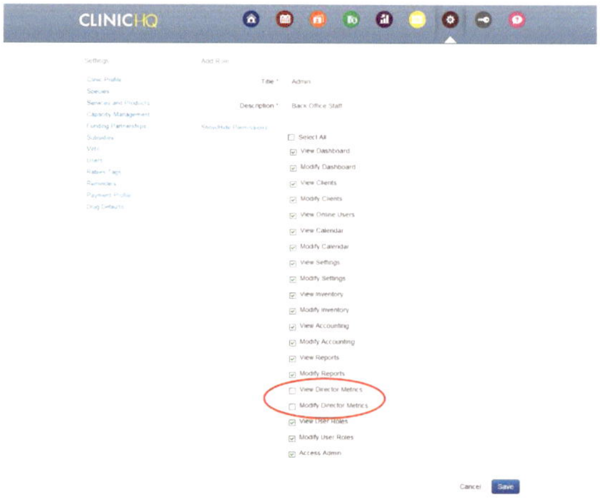

1. Click on <Settings> Icon
2. Click on blue <Users> link from the left hand main menu
3. The screen will default to <Users> tab under User Preferences screen
4. Click on <User Roles> tab to the right of the default <Users> tab
5. Click on <+Create Role> link in the upper right hand corner of the displayed grid
6. Enter Title and Description of the role (ex: Admin, Volunteer, Executive, etc.)
7. Select View/Hide Permissions to display a list of all of the items you want this user to either have or not have access to.

   Note: In the example above, this Admin role has access to all functions, except the

Executive Director Metrics.

8. Check the boxes to give access to each function, or click the select all box if no exclusions
9. Click the <Save> button at the bottom to create this role.

Create New User

1. Click on <Settings> Icon
2. Click on blue <Users> link from left hand main menu
3. Click the <+Create User> link in the upper right hand corner of the generated grid
4. Enter new user's first and last name
5. Enter clinic e-mail address and user name. These will be the same.
6. Choose user <Role> from the drop down menu (ex: Like the Admin role you created in the last section)
7. Make sure status is set to <Active>
8. Click blue <Setup User> button at the bottom to create the profile
9. New user will then be sent an e-mail with a link to set up their password

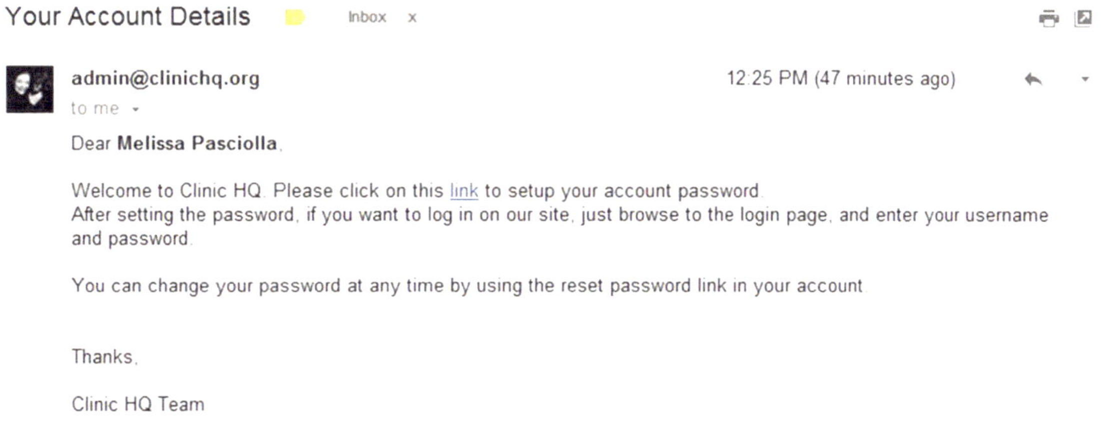
Your Account Details Inbox x

admin@clinichq.org 12:25 PM (47 minutes ago)

to me

Dear **Melissa Pasciolla**,

Welcome to Clinic HQ. Please click on this link to setup your account password.
After setting the password, if you want to log in on our site, just browse to the login page, and enter your username and password.

You can change your password at any time by using the reset password link in your account

Thanks,

Clinic HQ Team

Set Rabies Tag Allotments

Let Clinic HQ keep up with your rabies tag allotments for you. Here's how to set it up!

1. Click on <Settings> Icon
2. Click on blue <Rabies Tags> link from the left hand main menu
3. Choose the manufacturer of your clinic's rabies vaccine from the drop down menu
4. Choose Rabies 1-Year from the <Clinic Item> drop down menu
5. Enter the starting and ending tag numbers for the allotments on hand
6. Enter expiration date for the allotment
7. Enter the next tag number in line at your clinic from that allotment in <Next Tag Number> field
8. Repeat these steps to set your 3-Year Rabies allotment
9. Click the blue <Save> button to complete the setup

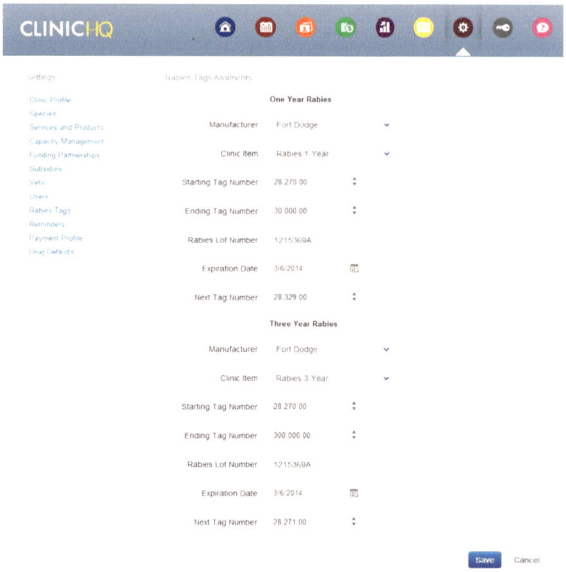

Create Client Reminders

There is evidence to support the fact that sending reminders to clients greatly reduces the number of no-shows for any business. That being said, Clinic HQ has implemented three options for your clinic to send reminders to your clients! Note: This is an additional service with some additional cost, but e-mail reminders are free. If call and sms (text) reminders are grayed out, and you cannot input values, then your clinic has opted out of this service.

1. Click on the <Settings> Icon
2. Click on blue <Reminders> link from the left hand main menu
3. Click <+Create Reminder> in the upper left hand corner of the Reminder Settings screen
4. Select call, sms (text), or e-mail as the <Reminder Type>

   Note: You will need to set up a reminder for all three types if they are enabled.
5. Select client type

   Note: You can choose to only send to public client or you can set up both types.
6. Check box to <Use this reminder for setting appointment confirmation>
7. Enter how many days before the appointment you would like the first reminder sent
8. Enter how many days before the appointment you would like the second reminder sent

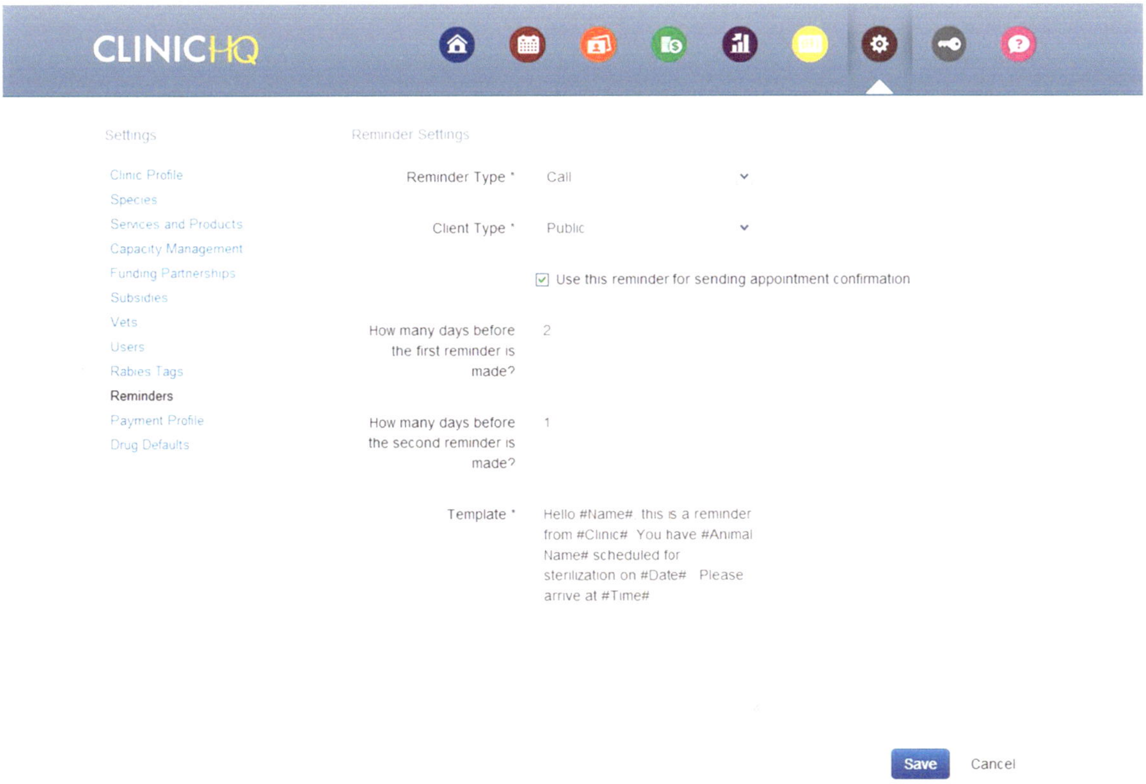

9. Enter the template that will be used for this particular reminder. (Examples Below)
10. Click <Save> to add this new type of reminder
11. Repeat this process to add all other types of reminders

Template Examples

- SMS (Text) Template For Public Client:

  Hello #Name#, this is a reminder from #Clinic#. You have #AnimalName# scheduled for sterilization on #Date#. Please arrive at #Time#.

- Call Template for Volume Client:

  Hello #Name#, you have #AnimalNumber# scheduled for sterilization on #Date#. Please give us a call and confirm your actual numbers. Thank you.

- Email Template for Public Client:

  Hello #Name#, this is a reminder from #Clinic#. You have #AnimalName# scheduled for sterilization surgery on #Date#. Please arrive at #Time#. Remember to withhold food after midnight the night before surgery, but water is ok. If your animal is under 4 months they can have food and water up to 2 hours before surgery. Please call if you have any other questions or concerns prior to your pet's surgery date. Thank you.

  Note: Your template can say whatever you wish. For example, if your clinic is difficult to find, you can include driving directions. Don't forget to use # on both sides of specific client information.

Chapter 7

User Preferences

Keep your clinic and client information confidential with Clinic HQ's security settings. Reset your password often to protect your profile, and always log out when Clinic HQ is not in use.

- Reset Password
- Log out of Clinic HQ

Reset Password

1. Click on <User Preferences> Icon
2. A menu will drop down below the <User Preferences> Icon
3. Choose <Change Password>

4. Key in your old password
5. Key in your new password twice
6. Click the <Submit> button to apply the change

Log out of Clinic HQ

1. Click on <User Preferences> Icon
2. A menu will drop down below the <User Preferences> Icon
3. Select the <Logout> option

Chapter

8

Community

Community: More than a Help Section

- Frequently Asked Questions
- Written Step by Step Tutorials
- Video Tutorials

Frequently Asked Questions

Browse our FAQ section of clinic HQ with a few clicks of your mouse. If you have a question about it, most likely someone else has as well. We will be constantly updating this part of the site with our most recent client feedback, so you won't have to go far to get the answers that you need!

This will be an ever evolving section of Clinic HQ.
Check in regularly to see our newest updates and latest features!

Written Step by Step Tutorials

Get the same helpful guidance we have provided in this manual in our Community section of Clinic HQ. Convenient, easy to follow steps for all major functions of the program can be found here.

Video Tutorials

For you visual learners, we will upload video tutorials to the site regularly. Browse our videos to get a quick lesson on specific functions of Clinic HQ!

Made in the USA
Las Vegas, NV
03 November 2026

57423048R00057